W9-DGC-999

The Relative Effectiveness of 10 Adolescent Substance Abuse Treatment Programs in the United States

Andrew R. Morral, Daniel F. McCaffrey,

Greg Ridgeway, Arnab Mukherji,

Christopher Beighley

Prepared for the Substance Abuse and Mental Health Services Administration,
Center for Substance Abuse Treatment

Drug Policy Research Center

A JOINT ENDEAVOR WITHIN RAND HEALTH
AND RAND INFRASTRUCTURE, SAFETY, AND ENVIRONMENT

The research described in this report was carried out under the auspices of the Drug Policy Research Center, a joint endeavor of RAND Infrastructure, Safety, and Environment (ISE) and RAND Health.

Library of Congress Cataloging-in-Publication Data

The relative effectiveness of 10 adolescent substance abuse treatment programs in the U.S. / Andrew R. Morral ... [et al.].
   p. cm.—(TR ; 346)
   Includes bibliographical references.
   ISBN 0-8330-3916-4 (pbk. : alk. paper)
   1. Youth—Substance use—United States. 2. Substance abuse—Treatment—United States. 3. Substance abuse—United States—Prevention. I. Morral, Andrew R. II.Title: Relative effectiveness of eleven adolescent substance abuse treatment programs in the U. S. III. Series: Technical report (Rand Corporation) ; 346.

HV4999.Y68R45 2006
616.86'0608350973—dc22

2006007643

The RAND Corporation is a nonprofit research organization providing objective analysis and effective solutions that address the challenges facing the public and private sectors around the world. RAND's publications do not necessarily reflect the opinions of its research clients and sponsors.

Published 2006 by the RAND Corporation
1776 Main Street, P.O. Box 2138, Santa Monica, CA 90407-2138
1200 South Hayes Street, Arlington, VA 22202-5050
4570 Fifth Avenue, Suite 600, Pittsburgh, PA 15213
RAND URL: http://www.rand.org/
To order RAND documents or to obtain additional information, contact
Distribution Services: Telephone: (310) 451-7002;
Fax: (310) 451-6915; Email: order@rand.org

Preface

Each year, substance abuse treatment programs in the United States record approximately 150,000 admissions of youths under the age of 18. Nevertheless, little is currently known about the effectiveness of the types of community-based services typically available to youths and their families. Recognizing the need for better information on the effectiveness of adolescent treatment services, the Substance Abuse and Mental Health Services Administration, Center for Substance Abuse Treatment (SAMHSA/CSAT) established the Adolescent Treatment Models (ATM) program. ATM grants were available to established adolescent treatment programs with at least suggestive evidence of effectiveness. These grants supported an independent, longitudinal evaluation of the client outcomes. Eleven such studies were funded in 1998 and 1999, each of which used parallel data collection instruments and study designs.

When the ATM studies were nearly complete, CSAT invited teams of researchers to examine whether evidence of treatment effectiveness was present in the collected longitudinal data. Analysis teams approached the problem of identifying treatment effects using a range of methods. This report describes RAND Corporation's approach to this problem, and our findings concerning the relative effectiveness of the 11 programs evaluated under ATM. This work was conducted in consultation with the ATM investigators who collected the data, and with other teams of investigators selected by SAMHSA/CSAT to conduct analyses with the same objective, but using different case-mix adjustment methods.

This report should be of interest to professionals with an interest in substance abuse treatment effectiveness, treatment evaluation methods, and risk or case-mix adjustment. It extends RAND's ongoing research on the effectiveness of community-based treatments for adolescents. Related publications from this line of RAND research include:

- Bluthenthal, R., Riehman, K. S., Jaycox, L. H., and Morral, A. R. (in press). Perspectives on therapeutic treatment from adolescent probationers. *Journal of Psychoactive Drugs.*
- Jaycox, L. H., Morral, A. R., and Juvonen, J. (2003). Mental health and medical problems and service utilization among adolescent substance abusers. *Journal of the American Academy of Child and Adolescent Psychiatry, 42,* 311–318.
- McCaffrey, D. F., Ridgeway, G., and Morral, A. R. (2004). Propensity score estimation with boosted regression for evaluating causal effects in observational studies. *Psychological Methods, 9,* 403–425.

- Morral, A. R., Jaycox, L. H., Smith, W., Becker, K., and Ebener, P. (2002). An evaluation of substance abuse treatment services provided to juvenile probationers at Phoenix Academy of Lake View Terrace. In S. J. Stevens and A. R. Morral (Eds.), *Adolescent Substance Abuse Treatment in America: Exemplary Models from a National Evaluation Study.* New York: Haworth Press.
- Morral, A. R., McCaffrey, D. F., and Chien, S. (2003). Measurement of adolescent drug use. *Journal of Psychoactive Drugs, 35,* 301–309.
- Morral, A. R., McCaffrey, D. F., and Ridgeway, G. (2004). Effectiveness of community-based treatment for substance abusing adolescents: 12-month outcomes from a case-control evaluation of a Phoenix academy. *Psychology of Addictive Behaviors, 18,* 257–268.
- Orlando, M., Chan, K., and Morral, A. R. (2003). Retention of court-referred youths in residential treatment programs: Client characteristics and treatment process effects. *American Journal of Drug and Alcohol Abuse, 29,* 337–357.
- Riehman, K. S., Bluthenthal, R., Juvonen, J., and Morral, A. R. (2003). Exploring gender differences among adolescents in treatment: Findings from quantitative and qualitative analyses. *Journal of Drug Issues,* Fall, 865–896.
- Schell, T., Orlando, M., and Morral, A. R. (2005). Dynamic effects among patients' treatment needs, beliefs, and utilization: A prospective study of adolescents in drug treatment. *Health Services Research,* 40, 1128–1147.
- Stevens, S. J., and Morral, A. R. (Eds.). (2003). *Adolescent Substance Abuse Treatment in the United States: Exemplary Models from a National Evaluation Study.* New York: Haworth Press.

The RAND Drug Policy Research Center

This study was carried out under the auspices of the Drug Policy Research Center, a joint endeavor of RAND Infrastructure, Safety, and Environment and RAND Health. The goal of the Drug Policy Research Center is to provide a firm, empirical foundation on which sound drug policies can be built, at the local and national levels. The center's work is supported by The Ford Foundation, other foundations, government agencies, corporations, and individuals.

This research was conducted within RAND Infrastructure, Safety, and Environment (ISE), a unit of the RAND Corporation. The mission of RAND Infrastructure, Safety, and Environment is to improve the development, operation, use, and protection of society's essential physical assets and natural resources and to enhance the related social assets of safety and security of individuals in transit and in their workplaces and communities.

Questions or comments about this report should be sent to the project leader, Andrew Morral (Andrew_Morral@rand.org). Information about the Drug Policy Research Center is available online (www.rand.org/multi/dprc/). Inquiries about Drug Policy Research Center projects should be made to the Center's Co-Directors, Peter Reuter (Peter_Reuter@rand.org) and Rosalie Pacula (Rosalie_Pacula@rand.org).

Inquiries regarding RAND Infrastructure, Safety, and Environment may be directed to its director:

Debra Knopman, Vice President and Director
ISE
RAND Corporation
1200 South Hayes Street
Arlington, VA 22202-5050
703-413-1100, x5667

The opinions expressed here are those of the authors and do not reflect official positions of the government.

Contents

Figures

Tables

Summary

Each year, substance abuse treatment programs in the United States record approximately 150,000 admissions of youths under the age of 18. Nevertheless, little is known about the effectiveness of the types of community-based services typically available to youths and their families. Recognizing the need for better information on the effectiveness of adolescent treatment services, the Substance Abuse and Mental Health Services Administration, Center for Substance Abuse Treatment (SAMHSA/CSAT) established the Adolescent Treatment Models (ATM) program. ATM grants were available to established adolescent treatment programs with at least suggestive evidence of effectiveness. These grants supported an independent, longitudinal evaluation of the client outcomes. Eleven such studies were funded in 1998 and 1999, each of which used parallel data collection instruments and study designs (see Stevens & Morral, 2003, for discussion of the 11 programs and each site's study design).

One of CSAT's program goals for the ATM projects was to establish whether any of the selected programs produce especially good client outcomes. However, to draw conclusions about the relative effectiveness of the ATM programs, it is probably not sufficient to simply compare the outcomes of youths at each program. Instead, some allowance must be made for the possibility that the youths treated at each program may not be identical. Specifically, programs may treat youths that differ with respect to how hard they are to treat or how great a risk of poor outcomes they present, in which case a simple comparison of outcomes or change in problems over time would not properly establish the relative effectiveness of the programs.

Because there are different approaches to case-mix adjustment that might yield different conclusions on the effectiveness of the ATM programs, CSAT decided to have the longitudinal data collected at the ATM programs subjected to several case-mix adjusted analyses of the relative effectiveness of the studied programs, each using a different approach, but examining a similar set of outcomes.

RAND's approach to examining the relative effectiveness of the 11 programs is designed to answer the question, "Will youths representative of those entering Program X have better outcomes if they receive treatment at Program X, rather than at one of the other studied programs?" This approach considers the possibility that programs may be most effective for the types of youths they typically serve. That is, programs may have adapted their interventions to optimally address the service needs of their treatment populations.

Data for the analyses presented in this report come from the 11 ATM studies. In each, all adolescent admissions were invited to participate in a longitudinal survey consisting of a baseline interview, and periodic follow-up interviews, including a 12-month post-admission assessment. All cases successfully interviewed at 12 months, as of March 2002, are included in the present analyses. This represents over 90 percent of the original baseline sample.

The substance abuse treatment programs for adolescents evaluated under ATM include three long-term residential (LTR) facilities (Dynamic Youth Community, Inc., in New York; Phoenix Academy of Los Angeles; and Thunder Road in Oakland), four short-term residential (STR) facilities (La Cañada in Tucson; Mountain Manor in Baltimore; Our Youth Our Future in Shiprock, New Mexico; and Thunder Road in Oakland), and four outpatient (OP) programs (Chestnut Health Systems in Bloomington, Illinois; Epoch Counseling Center in Baltimore County; Teen Substance Abuse Treatment in Maricopa County, Arizona; and The Village in Miami). Because of the small number of cases available for analysis at one ATM outpatient program, treatment effect estimates were not calculated for it.

In addition to the 263 LTR, 594 STR, and 404 OP cases followed under ATM at these 11 programs, an additional 128 LTR cases and 156 OP cases were also included in the ATM study and were available for inclusion in the present study as comparison cases. These cases came from a range of different community-based programs, which are not evaluated in this report.

Because this report is designed to examine whether there is any evidence of relative treatment effects, rather than to suggest that one or another treatment program is superior to others, we have obscured the identity of programs in the results section by referring to them as Programs A through J, designations assigned randomly within level of care.

Case-Mix Adjustment Approach

Our estimates of the causal effect of going to a particular facility as opposed to any other facility within the same level of care uses a case-mix adjustment approach in which weights are used to upweight eligible comparison cases most comparable to the treatment group cases, and down-weight those least comparable. The weights were chosen to maximize the similarity of the distributions for the target and comparison group cases on 86 control variables collected at treatment admission. Specifically we use propensity score weights estimated using the 86 control variables and a generalized boosting model (GBM). McCaffrey, Ridgeway, and Morral (2004) provide additional details on GBM propensity score weighting to estimate causal effects.

The pretreatment control variables used to perform the case-mix adjustment were drawn from the data collection instrument used in each ATM evaluation, the Global Appraisal of Individual Needs (GAIN; Dennis, 1999). The 86 GAIN items selected as control variables were identified by the GAIN's developer as operationalizing the American Society of Addiction Medicine (ASAM) Patient Placement Criteria (Mee-Lee, Shulman, Fishman, Gastfriend, and Griffith, 2001). ASAM patient placement criteria represent the best available empirical evidence and clinical judgment about the factors most important for determining patient placement and treatment needs. These variables concern substance use problems and severity; types, frequencies and histories of substances used; substance abuse, mental health, and physical health treatment histories and need; and many other potential risk factors (see Tables A.1 through A.4 in the appendix for a complete list of control variables).

Case-Mix Adjustment Results

Before adjusting comparison groups using propensity score weights, every treatment program was found to have cases that differed significantly from its respective comparison cases on many pretreatment risk factors. This shows that unadjusted comparisons of program outcomes, even within level of care, are likely to conflate true treatment effects with outcome differences attributable to outcome differences expected for cohorts exposed to different risks.

Propensity score weights greatly reduced the differences between control variable distributions. Indeed, satisfactory equivalence between treatment and comparison groups on the 86 pretreatment control variables was achieved for 4 of the 10 programs (B, G, H, and I), meaning that between-group differences on these pretreatment variables were no larger than would be expected had the same cases been randomly assigned to groups of equivalent size. Weighting was not sufficient to balance all pretreatment variables for Programs A, C, D, E, F, and J, meaning that at least one of the 86 variables showed group differences after weighting that were larger than would be expected had groups been formed through random assignment. For these programs, we took additional steps to ensure that outcome comparisons adjust for the remaining pretreatment group differences. Specifically, we included all such unbalanced variables as covariates in a weighted analysis of covariance (ANCOVA) model of treatment effects associated with these programs.

Using the derived propensity score weights, we estimated each program's relative treatment effects on six outcome measures assessed 12 months after treatment entry: (1) recovery, a dichotomous measure indicating the youth is free in the community and not using drugs, (2) substance problems, (3) substance use frequency, (4) illegal activities, (5) emotional problems, and (6) days in a controlled environment (like detention or a residential treatment program).

Results of the treatment effect estimates, by program, showed that across the 60 program and outcome pairs, only 11 significant relative treatment effects were observed. Moreover, many of the estimated effects were small. For instance, more than half of the estimated effects for substance abuse problems and substance abuse frequency were between −0.1 and 0.1.

Only five of the significant differences indicated treatment effects superior to those found in comparison sites. This scarcity of detectable positive relative treatment effects suggests that after controlling for pretreatment differences, the 12-month outcomes among the ATM programs differed by an amount too small to detect given the statistical power of our analyses.

The presence of six significant and negative effect sizes is also surprising but requires some caveats. First, half of these effects are for a single outcome variable, emotional problems. The relationship of this outcome to other traditional substance abuse treatment outcomes is not entirely clear. It could be argued, for instance, that some emotional distress might be an expected correlate of abstinence from the substances previously used to medicate those problems. Similarly, a fourth apparently negative effect size is the finding that Program C is associated with increased days in a controlled environment. However, in the context of an LTR program designed to treat youths for a year or more, this apparently inferior outcome might actually be due to the program's differential success retaining youth in the controlled environment of treatment, a seemingly beneficial effect. More difficult to explain is the negative effect size of Program E on recovery and of Program H on illegal activities, the latter of which also benefited from a particularly good case-mix adjusted comparison group.

Implications

When considering these 86 important pretreatment measures, the various programs appear to be serving distinctly different populations. Before weighting there were large and significant differences between every target program and its corresponding comparison programs. These differences were often for clearly important variables such as pretreatment substance use and the use of needles and opiates. Weighting by the propensity scores removes many of these differences but after weighting, several target programs continued to differ from their comparison group on potentially important risk factors.

The large differences between program clients resulted in small effective sample sizes for the weighted comparison cases. Combined with the small sample sizes in several programs the result was limited power to detect what are typically considered small effects. The use of ANCOVA in the current context potentially reduced power even more. Moreover, while treatment on the treated effect estimated in this report produce more substantively interesting results, it also comes at the cost of less precision for the estimated comparison group mean and potentially less power. Hence, the price of aggressive case-mix adjustment to avoid biased estimates may be a reduction in power for detecting true differences. Interestingly, in many cases described in this report, weighting and the consequent reduction in effective sample size did not appear to be the limiting factor for power. Instead, the reductions in effective sample size caused by weighting were compensated for by improvements in estimate precision. Future analyses should seek to evaluate treatment effects using larger samples, or by improving power in other ways.

Not surprisingly given the limitations of our analyses, the evidence favoring a view that one or more of the programs is especially effective with its treatment population is not particularly strong. However, what is somewhat surprising is that the most consistently small effects are for direct measures of substance use, the substance use problems and frequency indices. Given that the case-mix adjustment perspective we adopted for these analyses was designed to detect treatment effects resulting from adaptations programs have made to the specific characteristics of the clients they typically serve, or to detect more general types of superiority, we expected to find greater differences in the substance use measure. The findings of this report are similar to those reported from the Cannabis Youth Treatment project (Dennis et al., 2004) and Project MATCH (Matching Alcoholism Treatment to Client Heterogeneity) (Project Match Research Group, 1997). Specifically, differential treatment effects are not found, even though programs are compared, in some cases, to interventions involving fairly minimal treatment.

The modest evidence of differential effectiveness found in this study also may result from examining relative, rather than absolute treatment effects. Relative treatment effects yield ambiguous results. For instance, our finding that almost all estimated effects for the substance-use measures were small and that no STR or OP program appears to be more effective than its comparison programs at reducing substance use or substance problems admits a number of different interpretations.

- If all programs had poor absolute treatment effects on these outcomes, we might expect no relative treatment effects.
- If all programs had very large, but equivalent, absolute treatment effects on these outcomes, we would similarly expect no relative treatment effects.
- If the comparison sample is drawn from some programs that are more effective and some that are less effective than the program being evaluated, we might expect to find no relative treatment effects.

Moreover, even if relative differences do exist, we might expect them to be smaller than the effects we would find when comparing treatment to a no-treatment alternative and our analyses might have less power to detect relative differences than they would to detect difference against a control condition that received no treatment.

The possibility that all programs were effective, thereby reducing the chances of noting differential or relative treatment effects is worth considering. The 11 programs evaluated under ATM were not a random sample of community-based substance abuse treatment programs for adolescents. In fact, they were selected by CSAT for evaluation because they were able to demonstrate some evidence of effectiveness. Thus, the outcomes these programs produced may well have been unusually good across all programs, thereby reducing the appearance of differential treatment effects.

Finally, our failure to find strong and persuasive evidence of treatment effectiveness could indicate that we were looking for that evidence in the wrong place. Large and significant treatment effects might exist for each evaluated treatment program, but these might be no longer detectable 12 months after treatment admission. McLellan et al. (2005) have argued, for instance, that for chronic, relapsing conditions like substance abuse, the treatment effects of interest are chiefly those observed during treatment. By analogy, they note that treatments for other chronic conditions, like diabetes or schizophrenia, are typically evaluated in terms of symptom management during treatment, not by whether or not such benefits remain detectable long after treatments are withdrawn.

Whereas this argument has considerable appeal for treatment of adult chronic substance abusers, the applicability to adolescent substance abusers, many of whom appear to be in the early stages of substance abuse, is not yet well established. Clearly parents and other stakeholders would like to identify treatments that have long-lasting effects, making the evaluation of 12-month outcomes for adolescent treatments a valid, if nevertheless unpromising, enterprise.

In the absence of widely accepted and suitably specific quality-of-care indicators for adolescent substance abuse treatment, SAMHSA and many states are now exploring the use of outcomes-based performance measurement systems. The results from this study highlight a number of challenges to this plan and suggest strategies that should be considered in these and other efforts to understand treatment effects among individual programs, types of programs, or geographic regions.

Case-Mix Adjustment Is Important

The risk profiles of clients at different programs are quite variable. As a result, especially good or bad client outcomes may not reflect the performance of the treatment program, so much as the risk profiles of the clients it serves. Until the outcomes of comparable youths are compared, the relative effectiveness of different programs or groups of programs cannot be established. Similarly, if a program's client population changes over time, then comparisons of outcomes over time may not correspond to changes in that program's effectiveness. Finally, if risk profiles of clients differ by state, then comparisons of state treatment outcomes that fail to properly adjust for these differences are likely to be misleading.

Case-Mix Adjustment Is Not Enough

Even if the risk profiles of youths entering different programs were identical, this report highlights several ways in which valid conclusions about the effectiveness of different treatment programs may be difficult to draw from outcomes data. For instance, problems for interpretation arise when the proportion of cases providing follow-up data differs across programs. Thus, among the ATM programs, one had substantially lower rates of follow-up than the others, but the outcomes that were observed for this program appeared to be especially good. If those who are not followed up differed systematically from those who are, the outcomes for this program may be substantially more biased than those for the other ATM programs. Moreover, these are biases that may well be uncorrectable through, for instance, attrition weights, since the factors leading to study attrition may concern influences that occur long after the baseline assessment, such as nonresponsiveness to treatment. This suggests the need to ensure uniformly high rates of outcomes collection across programs.

Another challenge to the interpretation of outcomes concerns the high rates of institutionalization at follow-up observed in the ATM sample. When large proportions of cases are in controlled environments, many of the most important substance abuse treatment outcome measures are difficult to interpret. Thus, for instance, low levels of crime, drug use, and drug problems would ordinarily be viewed as a good outcome, but not if it reflects high rates of incarceration for a program's clients. Moreover, if programs from different geographic regions are compared, then differences in institutionalization rates cannot necessarily be attributed to treatment program effects. Instead, they might reflect differences in regional laws or law enforcement, the availability of inpatient services, or other community differences.

Indeed, community differences in resources, available support, opportunities, drug problems, and other characteristics may all influence the outcomes of youths in those communities, creating a significant confound for trying to establish effects specific to treatment programs on the basis of client outcomes, when those programs exist in different communities.

Each of these considerations suggest that even if case-mix adjustment is planned for outcomes-based performance measurement, valid conclusions about program performance may not be derivable from large-scale outcomes-monitoring systems.

Program Differences May Be Small

In this report, no program was found to consistently outperform any other, across outcomes. Indeed, few program differences were noted on any outcome, even though 70 percent of these analyses had sufficient power to detect effect sizes of 0.40 or greater. If differences in program effectiveness are generally small, this means that in order to detect performance differences, the outcomes of larger numbers of cases must be assessed before sufficient data is available to draw desired inferences. Since some programs see only small numbers of cases, and since the collection of outcomes data is often expensive, this finding has important implications for the feasibility of using outcomes to assess differences in the performance of individual programs.

Outcomes-Based Performance Measurement May Be Impractical

Many of the challenges described above raise important questions about the feasibility of producing valid treatment performance information from large-scale outcomes-based performance measurement efforts. This suggests that a more fruitful approach to performance measurement might be to invest more effort into identifying quality of care indicators for adolescent substance abuse treatment programs.

Acknowledgments

The research presented in this report owes thanks to the Adolescent Treatment Models (ATM) study investigators and their staffs who collected data on youths treated at the 11 programs. The investigators, who also provided valuable feedback at every stage of this study, are Robert Battjes, Mike Dennis, Marc Fishman, Susan Godley, Howard Liddle, Patricia Perry, Patricia Shane, Sally Stevens, Candice Sabin, and Tim Kinlock. We also thank Terry Schell of the RAND Corporation for reviewing a draft of this report. Finally, we thank Randy Muck, at the Center for Substance Abuse Treatment (CSAT), whose vision for the ATM study and other adolescent treatment investigations has dramatically improved what is known about adolescent treatment and its effectiveness.

In addition to the CSAT contract directly supporting the development of this report (270–2003–00006–0002, Westat prime), the work described here builds on other studies funded by a CSAT grant (KD1 TI11433) and by grants from the National Institute on Drug Abuse (R01 DA017507, R01 DA015697, R01 DA016722). Any errors remaining in the report are the responsibility of the authors.

Abbreviations

ANCOVA	Analysis of Covariance
ASAM	American Society of Addiction Medicine
ATM	Adolescent Treatment Models
ATT	average treatment effect on the treated
Days CE	days in a controlled environment during the past 90
CHS	Chestnut Health Systems
CSAT	Center for Substance Abuse Treatment
DSM-IV	*Diagnostic and Statistical Manual of Mental Disorders* (4th ed.)
EATT	expected average treatment effect on the treated
EPI[a]	Emotional Problems Index
GAIN	Global Appraisal of Individual Needs (survey)
GBM	Generalized Boosting Models
IAI[a]	Illegal Activities Index
ISE	Infrastructure, Safety, and Environment
KS	Kolmogorov-Smirnov (test statistic)
LTR	long-term residential (level of care)
MATCH	Matching Alcoholism Treatment to Client Heterogeneity
MAXCE	maximum days in a controlled environment
MDFT	Multidimensional Family Therapy
OP	Outpatient (level of care)
OYOF	Our Youth Our Future
SAMHSA	Substance Abuse and Mental Health Services Administration
SFI[a]	Substance Frequency Index
SOMMS	State Outcomes Measurement and Management System
SPI[a]	Substance Problems Index
STR	short-term residential (level of care)
TSAT	Teen Substance Abuse Treatment

[a] In this report we use the abbreviations for GAIN variables that correspond to the variable names in the Mar2002_CombineVmf dataset. The standard variables names for the GAIN have changed since this dataset was created, and the current names for the variables used in this report are: Emotional Problem Scale (EPS) for EPI; Illegal Activity Scale (IAS) for IAI; Substance Frequency Scale (SFS) for SFI; and Substance Problem Scale (SPS) for SPI.

CHAPTER ONE

Introduction

Each year, substance abuse treatment programs in the United States record more than 150,000 admissions of youths under the age of 18. Yet despite the widespread use of these treatment services by youths, little is known about their effectiveness. Although several studies suggest that novel or specialized approaches may be effective for youths (e.g., Azrin et al., 1994; Friedman, 1989; Henggeler, Melton, and Smith, 1992), community-based treatment centers like those at which most youths are treated have rarely been evaluated rigorously (Williams, Chang, and Addiction Centre Research Group, 2000; Winters, 1999).

Recognizing the need for better information on the effectiveness of community-based adolescent treatment programs, the Center for Substance Abuse Treatment, Substance Abuse and Mental Health Services Administration (CSAT/SAMHSA) established the Adolescent Treatment Models (ATM) program. ATM grants funded independent longitudinal evaluations of the outcomes of youths admitted to treatment programs that were able to provide at least suggestive evidence of effectiveness. In addition, ATM supported a detailed study of the cost of services delivered at each selected program, ethnographic case studies of youths' experiences in the selected programs, manual development to document the organization of services and their implementation at each program, and other goals (see Dennis et al., 2003).

In 1998, CSAT awarded the first ATM grants to three long-term residential (LTR) programs and three short-term residential (STR) programs. In 1998, five more grants were awarded, this time to an STR program and three outpatient programs (OP). Evaluation designs at each site were coordinated to facilitate cross-site analyses of the combined data. All 11 sites used the same core data collection instruments, each attempted to evaluate all youths admitted during the recruitment interval, and all interviewed youths around the time they were admitted to treatment and again 6 and 12 months later.[1]

Each grantee planned a site-specific outcome evaluation that used either a comparison group of youths who received a non-ATM treatment or one consisting of youths who received different interventions at the ATM program. The results from the site-specific studies will, therefore, address a range of questions specific to individual ATM programs. The results from these studies will not, however, clarify whether there are some ATM programs that appear to be achieving better youth outcomes than others.

---

[1] Some sites also conducted three- and nine-month interviews.

One of CSAT's program goals for the ATM projects was to establish whether any of the selected programs appears to be exemplary. However, in order to draw conclusions about the relative effectiveness of different ATM programs, some allowance must be made for the possibility that the youths treated at each program may not be identical. Specifically, programs may treat youths that differ with respect to how hard they are to treat, in which case a simple comparison of outcomes or change in problems over time would not properly establish the relative effectiveness of the programs.

The problem of establishing relative treatment effects when services are provided to non-equivalent client populations is one that has been considered at length in health services research. Indeed, there are now several major approaches for statistically adjusting relative treatment effect estimates to account for differences in program case mix, which we will hereafter refer to as "case-mix adjustment" approaches.

Because there are different approaches to case-mix adjustment that might yield different conclusions on the effectiveness of the ATM programs, CSAT decided to have the longitudinal data collected at the ATM programs subjected to several case-mix adjusted analyses of the relative effectiveness of the studied programs, each using a different approach, but examining a similar set of outcomes. The RAND Corporation performed one of these case-mix adjusted analyses of the effectiveness of the ATM programs. This report describes the RAND approach and findings.

RAND's Case-Mix Adjustment Perspective

Depending on the perspective taken in any case-mix adjustment analysis, a number of different questions might be addressed.[2] For instance, we could seek answers to any of the following questions on the relative effectiveness of the ATM programs:[3]

- Would youths representative of those seen at all ATM programs be expected to have superior outcomes had they gone to a particular ATM program?
- Are there particular types of youth who would be expected to have superior outcomes if they were treated at particular ATM programs?
- Will youths representative of those entering Program X have better outcomes if they receive treatment at Program X rather than one of the other studied programs?

Although the differences may appear subtle they have important implications for the case-mix adjustment approach and the conclusions that can be drawn from them. Analyses adopting the first perspective could help determine which programs are most effective for the

---

[2]   The perspective we describe is really about comparing treatment outcomes across alternative programs. This is typically done as part of a quasi-experiment where treatment is self-selected, and thus we refer to it as case-mix perspective.

[3]   These questions are all conditioned on the assumption that program effects are not necessarily constant across all youths. When treatment effects are not constant across youths, then we need to consider which subset of the population is the target of our inferences about program effects. If we assume constant effects, such as is done in classic linear regression adjustments, then only one effect is relevant, but our estimates could be very sensitive to the assumption of a constant effect.

average or typical youths. For our purposes, the first perspective, above, is clearly the least useful. ATM included only those youths admitted to one of a handful of purposively chosen programs, so the sample is not representative of youths seeking treatment generally. Moreover, since programs may be designed for the particular cases they treat, it would be inappropriate to evaluate them on the basis of some "average" youth who may be quite different from the program's treatment population.

The second perspective might be particularly useful for policymakers, referring agencies, and clients interested in identifying programs that will be most effective for a particular type of youths. For instance, probation departments might desire case-mix adjusted analyses adopting the second perspective to identify programs that are most effective for juvenile probationers.

The third perspective, and the one we adopt in this report, examines the possibility that programs may be most effective for the types of youths they typically serve. That is, programs may have adapted their interventions to optimally address the service needs of their treatment populations.

An advantage of our chosen case-mix perspective is that it does not constrain the results in such a way that if some programs do well, others must necessarily be found to do poorly. Indeed, it is perfectly possible that each program might be found to significantly outperform the others for cases like those typically treated by it. We believe this advantage outweighs the corresponding disadvantage that it may be difficult to determine whether there are some programs that are exemplary among the ATM cohort if all are found to be especially effective for cases like those they treat. If such a finding were to occur, it would suggest that treatment services need to be highly specialized and adapted to specific treatment populations. As such, simple conclusions about "the most effective" of the ATM programs would be inappropriate.

CHAPTER TWO

The ATM Programs

The 11 treatment programs selected by CSAT for evaluation include 3 long-term residential programs, four short-term residential programs, and 4 outpatient programs. Detailed descriptions of the program models, philosophies, and staffing may be found in Stevens and Morral (2003). Here we provide short descriptions of each program, highlighting their locations, structures, and general treatment mode.

In this section we provide the actual names of the programs, and the number of adolescent cases available from the program for evaluating its treatment effects. In later sections of this report, the order of programs is scrambled and their names are replaced by the letters A through I. By obscuring the identity of programs in the results sections, we have not attempted to, nor have we succeeded in, protecting the identity of the 11 programs (since these may be inferred by the client characteristics reported at each site). Instead, our intention is to focus attention on the questions of whether or not differential treatment effects can be detected, rather than on which program seems to be the best.

Since detailed descriptions of the characteristics of clients served at each program must be presented as part of the evaluation of the quality of the case-mix adjustments, we do not provide details here about the clients served by each program. Instead, tables describing client characteristics are presented in the Tables Appendix, and are linked not to actual names, but to letter identifiers.

Long-Term Residential Programs (LTR)

Dynamic Youth Community, Inc., is a treatment program in New York City for youths between the ages of 14 and 21 (Perry et al., 2003). Although the program includes outpatient phases, in this report we focus on 12-month follow-up outcomes associated with admission to the first phase of treatment. The first phase consists of a planned one-year stay in a 76-bed residential facility in upstate New York that uses a modified "therapeutic community" treatment model (see De Leon, 1999; Jainchill, 1997). For the treatment outcomes analyses presented in this report, data on 54 adolescents were available for assessing the effectiveness of this LTR treatment. The ATM study of Dynamic Youth Community was conducted by the New York State Office of Alcoholism and Substance Abuse Services (Patricia Perry, principal investigator).

Phoenix Academy of Los Angeles is also a modified therapeutic community treatment for adolescents, located in Lakeview Terrace, Los Angeles County (Morral et al., 2003). It is one of many Phoenix Academies operated by Phoenix House, a large, nonprofit treatment provider with programs around the United States. Youths between the ages of 13 and 17.5 enter this 150-bed residential program for a planned length of stay of 9 to 12 months. For this report, 152 ATM cases were available to assess program outcomes at this site. The ATM study of Phoenix Academy was conducted by RAND (Andrew Morral, principal investigator).

Thunder Road, a 50-bed residential treatment program in Oakland, California, is owned and operated by Adolescent Treatment Centers, Inc., a nonprofit service provider (Shane, Cherry, and Gerstel, 2003). Thunder Road offers both STR and LTR levels of care. Its LTR program offers a hybrid of therapeutic community, 12-step, and cognitive-behavioral treatment interventions, over a planned length of stay of 6 to 12 months. In the ATM study, 57 cases treated in Thunder Road's LTR program were available for outcomes analysis. The ATM study of Thunder Road was conducted by Public Health Institute (Patricia Shane, principal investigator).

Short-Term Residential Programs (STR)

La Cañada is an adolescent substance abuse treatment program in Tucson, Arizona, jointly developed by two nonprofit organizations, Arizona Children's Association and CODAC Behavioral Health Services (Stevens et al., 2003). La Cañada offers a "step-down" treatment model, beginning with 30 days of residential care for up to six boys and three girls, followed by two months of intensive outpatient aftercare. This phase is followed by two months of lower-intensity outpatient services. Residential treatment services for youths between the ages of 12 and 17 are guided by a milieu therapy philosophy and emphasize family therapy and individual and group counseling. In the ATM study, 166 cases treated at La Cañada were available for outcomes analysis. The ATM study was conducted by the University of Arizona—Services Research Office (Sally Stevens, principal investigator).

Mountain Manor Treatment Center offers a continuum of care to adolescents and young adults in Baltimore, Maryland (Fishman, Clemmey, and Adger, 2003). The ATM study evaluated only the STR treatment services at Mountain Manor, which are available to substance abusers between the ages of 11 and 20. The residential program offers a milieu therapy approach, with aspects of the treatment experience drawn from both medical models of addiction treatment and therapeutic community approaches. At the time of the ATM study, planned lengths of stay in this treatment track ranged from 10 to 60 days, with an average planned length of stay of 30 days. In the ATM study, 153 cases treated in Mountain Manor's STR program were available for outcomes analysis. This evaluation was conducted by Mountain Manor (Marc Fishman, principal investigator).

Our Youth Our Future (OYOF) is a 24-bed nonprofit residential treatment facility in Shiprock, New Mexico, serving substance-abusing youths, ages 12 to 19, from six major Native American tribes in reservation areas and reservation border towns in the four corners area of New Mexico. During the ATM study, the treatment program integrated culturally relevant experiences, practices, and philosophies about self-conduct with cognitive behavioral and bio-psychosocial treatment techniques (Stewart-Sabin and Chaffin, 2003). As such, this program provides an example of a treatment service explicitly designed for the target population of Native American youths. Therefore, we might expect that it is associated with better youth outcomes in this population than other programs not adapted to the needs and concerns of Native American youths. In the ATM study, 126 cases treated in OYOF were available for outcomes analysis. The ATM study of OYOF was conducted by the University of Oklahoma Health Sciences Center, Child Abuse and Neglect Research Office (Candice Sabin, principal investigator).

The fourth program classed as an STR treatment is Thunder Road in Oakland, which, as noted above, offers both STR and LTR treatment tracks for youths. Whereas their LTR treatment track has a planned length of stay of one year, the STR track has a planned length of stay of 30 to 50 days (Shane, Cherry, and Gerstel, 2003). The treatment philosophy, phases, and interventions are substantially similar for both the STR and LTR treatment tracks, with planned length of stay being the chief dissimilarity. Determination of which track youths enter is mainly controlled by payers, with private pay and private insurance opting for the STR track, and probation systems preferring the LTR track. In the ATM study, 149 youths treated in Thunder Road's STR track were available for outcomes analysis. The ATM study of Thunder Road was conducted by Public Health Institute (Patricia Shane, principal investigator).

Outpatient Programs (OP)

Chestnut Health Systems' (CHS) Bloomington, Illinois, outpatient adolescent treatment services are part of a continuum of CHS services that range from early intervention through residential interventions for youths between the ages of 12 and 18. The ATM study, however, examined the outcomes of a group of youths (n = 138) assigned using ASAM patient placement criteria to either the outpatient or intensive outpatient levels of care (Godley et al., 2003). Outpatient and intensive outpatient services are distinguished chiefly by the intensity of services provided; outpatient clients receive between 1 and 8 hours of services per week, whereas intensive outpatient cases receive between 9 and 12 hours per week. The CHS intervention approach blends concepts from Rogerian, behavioral, cognitive, and reality therapies, presented in individual and group counseling sessions. Cases entering both treatment tracks were considered to be OP cases for the purposes of the analyses in this report. The ATM evaluation was conducted by Chestnut Health System's research arm, Lighthouse Institute (Susan Godley, principal investigator).

Epoch Counseling Center, in Baltimore County, Maryland, is a private, nonprofit, service delivery component of Friends Research Institute, Inc. Epoch offers group-based outpatient adolescent treatment services to adolescents between the ages of 14 and 18, using a treatment approach that combines motivational interviewing and psychoeducational techniques with group and family counseling sessions (Battjes et al., 2003). For the ATM study, 157 youths were available to assess 12-month outcomes after admission to Epoch Counseling Center. The ATM evaluation was conducted by Friends Research Institute's Social Research Center (Robert Battjes, principal investigator).

Teen Substance Abuse Treatment (TSAT) in Maricopa County, Arizona, offers intensive outpatient services to adolescent substance abusers between the ages of 12 and 17 and their families (Stevens, Estrada et al., 2003). Treatment services consist of in-home individual and family counseling, using techniques drawn from cognitive-behavioral and family systems therapies. In addition, youths and their families participate in teen group therapy and multifamily group therapies. Planned duration of treatment is 90 days with over 9 hours of service provided weekly. In the ATM study, 97 youths treated at TSAT were available for outcomes analyses. The ATM study of TSAT was conducted by the University of Arizona—Services Research Office (Sally Stevens, principal investigator).

The Village, Inc. in Miami, Florida is a nonprofit substance abuse treatment program that offers both adult and adolescent outpatient treatment services. For the ATM study, the Village participated in an experimental evaluation of a version of Multidimensional Family Therapy (MDFT; Liddle et al., 2001) as an early intervention for young adolescents in the early stages of exhibiting substance abuse problems (Liddle et al., 2004). Specifically, youths between the ages of 11 and 15 were randomly assigned to MDFT or to group counseling sessions conducted twice per week for between 12 and 16 sessions. The ATM study of MDFT at the Village was conducted by the University of Miami School of Medicine (Howard Liddle, principal investigator). At the time data for the present report were collected, just 12 cases were available from the Village, too few to support valid inferences about program effects. Consequently, no outcomes analyses were performed for this program.

Whereas the sections above describe the programs selected by CSAT for evaluation, locally, some evaluation designs included collection of data on youths attending comparison programs. Thus, an additional 128 LTR cases and 156 OP cases were available for inclusion in the present study as comparison cases. These cases came from a range of different community-based programs that are not evaluated in this report.

CHAPTER THREE

Case-Mix Adjustment Approach

All of the ATM programs were associated with improvements in 12-month outcomes. Figure 3.1, for instance, shows pretreatment and 12-month substance use problems and substance use frequencies for each of the 10 programs examined in this report. On each measure, every program is associated with statistically significant improvements ($p < .01$). Whereas improvements like these are encouraging and have often been used to suggest the effectiveness of treatments, no such conclusions can be validly drawn from these results. For a treatment to be considered effective, we must demonstrate that youths who received that treatment would have had worse outcomes had they received alternative care (such as no treatment or treatment at a different facility). Because the pretreatment and 12-month follow-up data in Figure 3.1 provide no evidence concerning how these same youths might have done had they not received treatment, we cannot rule out the possibility that observed improvements result from factors other than treatment, such as normal maturation, regression to the mean, or history effects (Shadish, Cook, and Campbell, 2002).

Just as improvements cannot be attributed unequivocally to program effects, differences between programs in the extent of improvements also are not good indicators of the relative effectiveness of different programs. For instance, it might be tempting to judge Program C to be more effective than Program A, for instance, because it takes youths with more severe drug use and problems, and 12 months later they have much better outcomes than those of youths in Program A. Without additional information about other pretreatment differences between youths entering Program A and Program C, however, we cannot attribute these outcome differences to treatment effects, as opposed to pretreatment risk factors. For instance, if Program A primarily treats hard-core addicts who are at high risk for continued drug use and problems, whereas Program C treats youths with much better prognoses, then the differences observed in Figure 3.1 could be quite misleading.

To establish the effect of a treatment program, or its effect relative to that of another treatment program, we must compare outcomes of youths seen at the program to the outcomes of the same youths had they received a different treatment. Of course, the same group of youths cannot both be treated at a program and not treated there for comparison purposes. Instead, our estimate of the causal effect of going to a particular facility as opposed to any other facility within the same level of care uses a case-mix adjustment approach in which propensity score weights are used to upweight eligible comparison cases most similar to the treatment group cases and downweight those least similar. This procedure creates a synthetic comparison group

Figure 3.1
Pretreatment and 12-Month Follow-Up Substance Problems and Use Frequency by Program

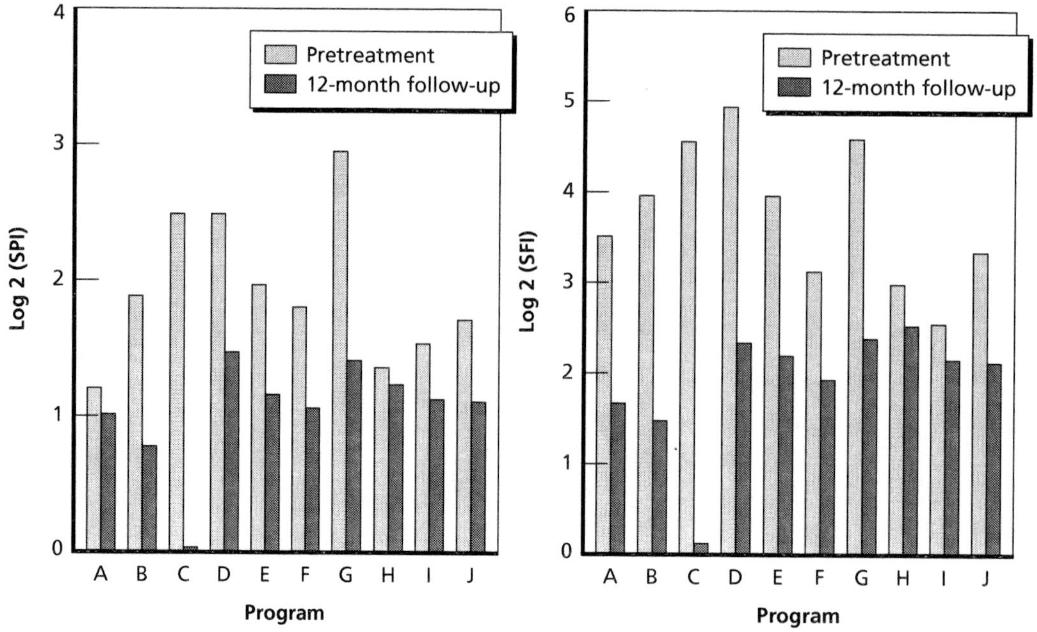

RAND *TR346-3.1*

with pretreatment characteristics similar to those in the treatment group. On the basis of these similarities, any differences in outcomes observed between groups must be attributable either to the treatment effects of interest, or to unobserved pretreatment characteristics that distinguish the groups.

In this section, we first define the causal effect we wish to estimate for each facility. We then describe the case-mix adjustment procedure used for estimating the effect of interest.

The Treatment Effect

As discussed above, our interest is in the relative treatment effect for each facility compared to other facilities providing a similar level of care. Because all cases in the study received some sort of care, treatment effects are the differential or relative effects of the various programs. However, we will typically use the terms "treatment effect" to refer to these differential effects to simplify presentation. We use the Rubin Causal Model (Holland, 1986) to define treatment effects. This model is premised on the idea that each individual has two "potential outcomes" at admission. The first is the adolescent's outcome if he or she receives treatment at the target facility. We denote this potential outcome with y_1. The second is the adolescent's outcome if he or she receives treatment at one of the other treatment facilities. We denote this potential outcome with y_0.[1] The relative treatment effect for the target facility is then the difference between these potential outcomes for each youth $(y_1 - y_0)$. Because the magnitude of these treatment effects can vary across youths, they should be thought of as an entire distribution of treatment effects. To summarize the effects of treatment at a facility, therefore, we may consider the average treatment effect across youths. As discussed above, however, we are not interested in a facility's effect on youths it will never treat. Hence we consider the average treatment effect among youths who are actually treated by the target facility. This effect is often referred to as the average treatment effect on the treated (ATT; Wooldridge, 2001).

We let T be an indicator variable for receiving treatment at the target facility: $T = 1$ if a youth receives treatment at the target facility, $T = 0$ otherwise. Every youth in the population will have one observable value of T depending on where he or she receives treatment and two potential but not necessarily observable outcomes, y_1 and y_0. We let $E(y_1 \mid T = t)$ denote the conditional expected value or mean of y_1, given a particular value of T. For example, $E(y_1 \mid T = 1)$ is the mean of the outcome after receiving treatment at the target facility for youths who receive treatment at that facility and $E(y_1 \mid T = 0)$ is the mean of the potential outcome after receiving treatment at the target facility for youths who receive care at the comparison programs. The means can be over differ groups if youths who enter the target program differ from other youths on pretreatment characteristics. However, for both groups, the expectation is for the potential outcome that results if the youths receive care at the target facility. The values might differ if there are preexisting differences among the youths who receive care at alternative facilities. We define $E(y_0 \mid T = t)$ and $E(y_1 - y_0 \mid T = t)$ analogously. Using this notation we define the treatment effect of interest to our study:

$$ATT = E(y_1 - y_0 \mid T = 1) = E(y_1 \mid T = 1) - E(y_0 \mid T = 1) \qquad (1)$$

ATT is defined as the difference of the conditional expected value of potential outcomes for youths treated at the target facility. It describes the target facility's effect on its client population. If all programs are particularly effective at treating their cases, then ATT could be positive for every program.

The treatment effect we consider is defined as the mean difference in potential outcomes. Treatment effects are not defined in terms of change scores or regression coefficients because they do not represent how the treatment has actually changed a youth's outcomes. Rather those quantities provide descriptions of growth or statistical models developed to estimate the causal effect. In particular, given that adolescents' drug use changes considerably over time and that treatment often follows periods of high use, we might expect to find that on average substance use declines from intake to the 12-month follow-up regardless of the treatment program a youth might enter or even if the youth received no treatment at all. Hence an overall decline in use cannot be attributed to a treatment effect, because it may occur whether or not youths' potential outcomes in treatment or not in treatment differ. If a treatment program results in greater changes than the youths' potential changes at other facilities, then we attribute this dif-

---

[1] The potential outcome depends on the alternative treatment facility at which the adolescent would receive treatment. We assume each youth would receive treatment at only one alternative facility and it is his or her outcome at this facility that constitutes y^0.

ferential change to the program's treatment effect. However, given a youth can have only one potential pretreatment outcome, differences in potential change scores are equal to differences in the potential outcomes at follow-up. Therefore causal effects are defined only in terms of the potential outcomes following treatment.

Estimating the Treatment Effect

Estimation of the treatment effect is complicated because we cannot observe both potential outcomes for the entire population. In fact, we can observe only a single potential outcome for each youth in a sample from the population. We observe y_1 when $T = 1$ for youths who received treatment in the target facility, and we observe y_0 when $T = 0$ for others. We have no direct observations of y_0 when $T = 1$, the outcome that would have happened to this subject treated at the target facility had they been treated at a comparison facility. Moreover, as noted above, if youths who receive treatment at the target facility differ systematically from other youths in ways that are associated with outcomes, then $E(y_0 \mid T = 1)$ will not equal $E(y_0 \mid T = 0)$, and simple summaries of our observed data will not provide an estimate of the desired treatment effect.

However, if we can assume that we observe control variables that fully describe any differences between youths receiving care at the target facility and those receiving care at other facilities, then case weights, w_i, can be constructed that alter the covariate distributions for the comparison group so that it matches that of the treatment group (Hirano, Imbens, and Ridder, 2003; McCaffrey, Ridgeway, and Morral, 2004). Therefore, these weights yield an unbiased estimate of the desired treatment effect:[2]

$$EATT = \frac{\sum\limits_{i=1}^{n} y_i t_i}{\sum\limits_{i=1}^{n} t_i} - \frac{\sum\limits_{i=1}^{n} y_i w_i (1 - t_i)}{\sum\limits_{i=1}^{n} w_i (1 - t_i)} \tag{2}$$

where n is the total number of youths in the study sample, t_i is the value of the treatment indicator for the ith study participant, y_i is the observed outcome value (i.e., y_i equals y_1 when $t_i = 1$ and y_1 when $t_i = 0$). The weights are the estimated conditional odds of receiving treatment at the target facility. That is

$$w_i = \frac{p(x_i)}{1 - p(x_i)} \tag{3}$$

---

[2] If the weights are estimated then the expected average treatment effect on the treated (EATT) is unbiased in large samples. See Hirano, Imbens, and Ridder (2003) for details.

where x_i denotes the vector of control variables and $\hat{p}(x_i)$ is the estimated conditional probability of receiving treatment for a youth with control variables equal to x_i, otherwise known as the propensity score (Rosenbaum and Rubin, 1983). Details on the estimator EATT can be found in McCaffrey, Ridgeway, and Morral (2004).

Statistical Methods

Propensity scores were estimated using generalized boosted regression, a data-adaptive, non-parametric, logistic regression procedure (GBM, generalized boosting models; Ridgeway, 1999, 2004). Specifically, 86 control variables collected at treatment admission (see Measures, Chapter 4) were used to predict t, the dichotomous treatment indicator that equals 1 if the youth received treatment in the target facility and 0 if he or she received treatment in another facility within the same level of care (LTR, STR, or OP). McCaffrey, Ridgeway and Morral (2004) provide additional details on using GBM to estimate propensity scores.[3]

The goal of the propensity score weighting is to make the covariate distributions for the comparison group comparable to those for the treatment group. Therefore, we evaluate the quality of our propensity score weights by whether there are differences in the treatment and weighted comparison covariate distributions that are greater than might be expected in a study in which these groups were constructed using random assignment. Differences in each control variables distribution between groups is assessed with the Kolmogorov-Smirnov (KS) test statistic. The KS statistic is a nonparametric measure defined as the largest absolute difference in the cumulative distribution functions of two samples. It ranges from 0, indicating that at no point do the distributions diverge, to 1, indicating no overlap between distributions. We estimate the probability that the observed maximum weighted KS statistic, across baseline control variables, would be found in a random assignment study with a randomization test. In the randomization test, new groups of a size equal to the target and unweighted (or weighted) control group samples are randomly drawn from the pooled target sample and unweighted (or weighted) comparison samples. After hundreds of such randomizations, we can estimate the distribution of maximum KS statistics expected across the control variables, given their unique covariance structure in the pooled sample.

Even if weighting is generally successful in removing pretreatment differences, some control variables might retain notable differences between the target and comparison samples after weighting. To account for these differences we include any such variables as covariates in a weighted analysis of covariance when estimating the adjusted treatment effect. Specifically, we include as a covariate in the treatment effect analysis any covariate with a weighted KS test that is significant at the 0.05 level (i.e., if the p-value for the KS test is less than 0.05).

---

[3] In their paper, McCaffrey, Ridgeway, and Morral suggest tuning the GBM model by selecting the number of iterations used in the GBM algorithm to minimize the average standardized absolute mean difference on the control variables used in fitting the propensity score model. For this report, we adopted a more demanding criterion. Namely, we tuned the GBM model by choosing the number of iterations to minimize the average Kolmogorov-Smirnov test statistic for the difference between treatment and comparison groups in the distributions of the control variables.

To highlight the effects of each step in this estimation procedure, we present in this report three estimated treatment effects: the unweighted estimate; the propensity score weighted estimate; and the weighted analysis of covariance estimates.

CHAPTER FOUR

Study Procedures

Sample Description

The sample used in the present analysis includes all available cases from the ATM study as of March, 2002, when the main analytic data file[1] was created by Chestnut Health Systems, the organization that served as the coordinating center for the ATM projects (Michael Dennis, principal investigator). Because we wish to examine treatment effects 12 months post-admission, the sample was restricted to just those 1,545 cases with completed 12-month assessments. This sample also excluded cases admitted to a continuing-care intervention that represented a new phase of care for clients who had been admitted to treatment more than a year earlier.

A small number of cases were admitted to their respective treatment programs less than 12 months prior to March 2002. Because these cases had no 12-month assessments in the dataset, they were excluded by design. Since we assume in this report that treatment effects are constant over the period of study, we can also assume that the exclusion of these cases introduces no bias into our treatment effect estimates. More problematic are those cases excluded because they were lost to follow-up. Such cases can be systematically different than those retained in the sample (Scott, 2004), so their exclusion may introduce bias. Although follow-up rates across the ATM studies were excellent overall, with 91 percent of all cases interviewed at 12 months, one site had a follow-up rate of just 71 percent. We will return later to the possible effects that this lower follow-up rate might have on that program's apparent relative treatment effects. With the exception of this program, no program had a follow-up rate lower than 86 percent, so restricting the sample to just those assessed at 12 months probably does not introduce substantial bias in our treatment effect estimates for those programs.

At each treatment program, all admissions were invited to participate in the study within seven days of their admission, using procedures approved by local Institutional Review Boards. All participants were volunteers who provided written informed assent, and for whom written consent was provided by a parent or guardian.

---

[1] The file is called Mar2002_CombineVmf.

Measures

Data collection included a baseline assessment, and follow-up assessments 6 and 12 months after their baseline interviews (some programs conducted additional follow-up assessments 3 or 9 months after admission). Data collection was conducted by local interviewers trained to criterion performance on the survey instrument used at every site, the Global Appraisal of Individual Needs (GAIN; Dennis, 1999) and its follow-up versions. The GAIN is a structured clinical interview collecting information in eight main topic domains (background, substance use, physical health, risk behaviors, mental health, environment, legal, vocational). The GAIN includes over 100 symptom, change score, and utilization indices that have good internal reliabilities and have been evaluated on large samples of adults and adolescents (Dennis et al., 2002, 2003, 2004; Dennis, Scott et al., 1999).

Outcome Measures

We consider six different outcome[2] measures for evaluating differences among the ATM facilities: recovery, substance problems, substance use frequency, illegal acts, emotional problems, and time in controlled environments (see Table 4.1).

Table 4.1
Twelve-Month Outcomes Used in Treatment Effect Analyses by Treatment Programs, After Transformation

Program		Recovery	Substance Problems		Substance Frequency		Illegal Actions		Emotional Problems		Cont. Envi't	
		%	mean	sd	mean	sd	mean	sd	mean	sd	mean	sd
LTR	A	0.246	1.013	1.388	1.627	1.937	0.381	0.171	0.303	0.174	40.875	36.182
	B	0.250	0.770	1.173	1.486	1.911	0.368	0.191	0.213	0.164	40.468	38.412
	C	0.185	0.029	0.171	0.116	0.675	0.245	0.105	0.150	0.108	77.941	29.454
	All LTR	0.266	0.764	1.171	1.258	1.845	0.361	0.183	0.221	0.169	45.118	38.898
STR	D	0.261	1.479	1.562	2.342	2.190	0.440	0.199	0.300	0.185	17.458	30.931
	E	0.169	1.155	1.377	2.190	1.961	0.434	0.216	0.216	0.151	25.677	37.086
	F	0.341	1.054	1.320	1.914	1.883	0.337	0.194	0.190	0.149	15.092	30.174
	G	0.315	1.408	1.494	2.384	2.020	0.425	0.206	0.274	0.193	13.825	27.136
	All STR	0.266	1.276	1.448	2.217	2.019	0.412	0.208	0.245	0.176	18.321	32.019
OP	H	0.217	1.241	1.226	2.528	1.792	0.445	0.213	0.220	0.176	9.396	23.599
	I	0.341	1.120	1.234	2.135	1.987	0.362	0.206	0.226	0.177	11.230	25.235
	J	0.216	1.111	1.256	2.110	1.886	0.378	0.208	0.157	0.138	22.088	32.431
	All OP											

NOTE: See text for discussion of how each measure has been transformed.

---

[2] The term "outcome" is misleading in the case of some youths in the long-term residential programs who have not yet left treatment by the 12-month follow-up assessment. For these youths, the 12-month interview collects what might better be referred to as an "interim outcome." Nevertheless, for simplicity, we have adopted the term "outcomes" for all cases.

Recovery is a dichotomous measure indicating that the youth is living in the community and experiencing few symptoms of substance use, abuse, or dependence. Specifically, recovery is 1 if the respondent is not in detention at the time of the interview, has not been in any other controlled environment for more than 15 of the last 90 days, and reports no symptoms of substance abuse or dependence in the past month.

Substance problems are measured using the GAIN's Substance Problem Index (SPI). The SPI is a 16-item count of self-reported symptoms of substance abuse and dependence experienced in the 30 days prior to the interview. Seven items from this index correspond to *Diagnostic and Statistical Manual of Mental Disorders* (4th ed.) (DSM-IV) criteria for dependence, and four for abuse (American Psychiatric Association, 1994). Five additional items assess other common symptoms of substance misuse. The SPI has shown good internal consistency (Cronbach alpha = .9) and test-retest reliability ($r = .7$) in prior research (Dennis et al., 2003; Dennis, Titus, et al., 2002; Godley et al., 2002). A base two log transformation is used to improve the distribution of this outcome.

Substance use frequency is assessed using the GAIN's Substance Frequency Index (SFI). The SFI takes the average of responses to seven GAIN items concerning the number of days in the past 90 during which there was: (1) reported use of alcohol, marijuana, cocaine or heroin, (2) use to intoxication, and (3) a failure to perform routine activities due to substance use. Like a "sources of income" scale, there is no expectation that a common factor contributes to the variance in each item, so inter-item reliability is neither expected nor assessed. Whereas the Chestnut version of this Index takes the average described above divided by 90, ours uses a base two log transformation to improve the variable's distribution.

The illegal activities outcome is assessed using the GAIN's Illegal Activities Index (IAI). The IAI is constructed by averaging three GAIN items (recency of illegal activities, days of illegal activities in the past 90, and days supporting self through illegal activities in the past 90) after transforming each to a 0 to 1 range. In the baseline sample of 1,582 ATM cases analyzed by Chestnut Health Systems in their Main Findings tables (Dennis, McDermeit, and Funk, 2002), the IAI was found to have good inter-item reliability (Cronbach alpha = .78). To improve the distribution of the IAI, we use a square root transformation.

We assess emotional problems at follow-up using the GAIN's Emotional Problem Index (EPI). The EPI averages seven GAIN items assessing the recency, frequency, and severity of psychological distress, after transforming each item to have a range of 0 to 1. In the ATM Main Findings Tables, the 1,582 ATM baseline cases demonstrated that the EPI had good internal reliability (Cronbach alpha = 0.80; Dennis, McDermeit, and Funk, 2002).

Finally, we assess time in a controlled environment using the GAIN's MAXCE (maximum days in a controlled environment) variable, which calculates the maximum number of days, in the past 90, in which the respondent reports being in any of several different types of controlled environments (e.g., inpatient psychiatric or medical hospitals, residential treatment facilities, juvenile halls or other criminal justice detention facilities, etc.) or on which the respondent reports either being in a controlled environment where they were not free to come and go as they please, or in which they could not use alcohol or drugs. Like a "sources of income" scale, there is no expectation that a common factor contributes to the variance in each item, so inter-item reliability is neither expected nor assessed.

Table 4.1 provides means and standard deviations for the outcome variables by program and level of care. Because recovery is dichotomous, only the percentage of the sample in recovery is provided. Differences in the means might not reflect differential treatment effects for programs or level of care, because these differences might result from differences in the pretreatment risk factors of the adolescent cohorts entering each program.

Baseline Control Variables

The GAIN-I contains over 1,000 items that could be used in a case-mix adjustment analysis. Nevertheless, ensuring that treatment and comparison groups have equivalent distributions on control variables that are irrelevant either to placement decisions or expected outcomes unnecessarily reduces the power of the outcomes analysis. Optimally, therefore, only those variables that are relevant to the treatment placement decision and to expected outcomes would be included as control variables in the case-mix adjustment analysis. These variables might be identified empirically or on theoretical or a priori grounds. For the analyses presented in this report, we adopt the latter approach. That is, a priori we selected GAIN items corresponding to the American Society of Addiction Medicine (ASAM) patient placement criteria (Mee-Lee et al., 2001). ASAM patient placement criteria represent the best available empirical evidence and clinical judgment about the factors most important for determining patient placement and treatment needs.

The GAIN has been developed to assist clinicians with patient placement decisions, so it includes items designed to operationalize the ASAM criteria. These include more than 80 items and measures assessing substance use problems and severity; types, frequencies and histories of substances used; substance abuse, mental health, and physical health treatment histories and need; schooling, employment, and criminal justice history; psychological, psychiatric, and spirituality measures; measures of problem behaviors, including risk behaviors, criminal behavior, violent and suicidal behavior, coping, and victimization; measures of family, peer, financial, and environmental support; stress; age, race, and gender; and other characteristics (see Tables A.1 through A.3 in the Tables Appendix for a complete list of control variables).

As this list demonstrates, the items and measures included as control variables are not only appropriate because they are identified by ASAM as relevant to placement decisions; they also represent the kinds of pretreatment characteristics we might expect to serve as risk and protective factors for various of the 12-month outcomes, so ensuring treatment and comparison group comparability on these items improves confidence that the case-mix adjusted treatment effect estimates are valid.

The 86 control variables included in the case-mix adjusted treatment effect estimates included in this report were selected from a larger list of 111 items identified by the GAIN's developer as operationalizing ASAM Patient Placement criteria (Dennis, personal communication, June 2004). Twenty-five of the larger set of items were excluded either because there was no variation in responses across the sample (e.g., items concerning recent delirium tremens, and youths' parenting behaviors), there was too much missing data due to sites not asking the questions (e.g., items concerning parental income and youth sexual risk), or the item or scale was added to the GAIN after the ATM study baseline interviews were conducted (e.g., strength self-efficacy, reasons for wanting to quit).

Surviving control variables had low rates of missingness. Nevertheless, missing values were imputed using a regression model hot-deck imputation procedure (Little and Rubin, 1987). Specifically, for a given variable with missing values, we modeled the expected value of the variable as a function of demographic characteristics, drug use history, psychological status, treatment history, legal history, and other control variables. Records were stratified into 10 sets by the percentiles of the predicted scores from this fitted model. For each observation with a missing value, a "donor" value was drawn at random from the records in the same predicted score stratum as the case with the missing value. This donor value served as the imputed value for the outcome. The variables were imputed sequentially, allowing variables imputed with more available data to be used in the imputation of variables with more missing data.

CHAPTER FIVE

Case-Mix Adjusted Comparison Samples

Before presenting case-mix adjusted treatment effects associated with each program, we first consider our success in creating weighted comparison groups with covariate distributions comparable to each of the target treatment groups.

KS statistics describing the dissimilarity between target and comparison programs before and after weighting are summarized in Table 5.1 (for details on comparability of each of the 86 control variables, see the Tables Appendix, which also includes unadjusted means and standard deviations for all control variables by facility). For example, we compared the distribution of each of the 86 pretreatment control variables of cases from Program A to the corresponding distribution of all other LTR cases, yielding 86 KS statistics. The largest of these 86 statistics was 0.587 (shown in the first row of Table 5.1), indicating that Program A youths differ substantially from non-program A youths on at least one of the 86 variables. The small p-value indicates that this value is significantly greater than would be expected if the same cases had

Table 5.1
Comparability of Target and Comparison Covariate Distributions Before and After Weighting: Summary Results

Program	Unweighted		Weighted	
	Max KS	p value	Max KS	p value
LTR				
A	0.587	<.01	0.329	<.01
B	0.337	<.01	0.167	0.62
C	0.668	<.01	0.481	<.01
STR				
D	0.316	<.01	0.306	<.01
E	0.380	<.01	0.316	<.01
F	0.925	<.01	0.441	<.01
G	0.446	<.01	0.182	0.68
OP				
H	0.302	<.01	0.190	0.15
I	0.345	<.01	0.193	0.10
J	0.388	<.01	0.259	<.01

been randomly assigned to equally large groups. Similarly, each of the other programs has maximum KS statistics larger than would be expected had the same cases been randomly assigned to groups, suggesting that programs within the same level of care are treating populations that differ substantially on at least one baseline covariate. In fact, as may be seen in Tables A.4 through A.14 (in the Tables Appendix), facilities within a level of care tend to treat youths with many different pretreatment characteristics. For Program A, for instance, Table A.4 reveals there were 57 variables with significant mean differences before weighting, 23 control variables had effect sizes greater than 0.5, and the average between group effect size was 0.42, a substantial average difference.[1]

Weighting greatly reduces the differences between covariate distributions, reducing the maximum KS statistic by nearly half, and reducing the number of large-effect size differences seen in Appendix Table A.4. Nevertheless, as is evident in Table 5.1, even these reductions are not sufficient to reduce Program A's maximum KS statistic to a magnitude that might be expected had groups been formed by random assignment.

These results suggest that we obtained comparison groups for four programs that appear to be very good: the largest KS statistics for Programs B, G, H, and I are all smaller than might be expected at least 10 percent of the time had groups been formed by random assignment rather than by natural selection processes. Furthermore, for each program nearly all the 86 KS statistics are very small and not statistically significant. Thus, for these programs we believe that differences between the program means and the weighted comparison means provide acceptable estimates of the program effects, without additional adjustments.

However, weighting was not sufficient for some programs to make the cases from the comparison programs comparable to the cases from the target program. Programs A, C, D, E, F, and J had at least one KS statistic among the 86 variables that was larger than would be expected had groups been formed through random assignment. For these programs, additional adjustment was attempted to control for these remaining differences. Thus, we include all variables with significant KS statistics (p < .05) as covariates in a weighted analysis of covariance (ANCOVA) model when estimating the program's treatment effects. Nevertheless, the failure of weighting to identify cases with similar covariate distributions suggests that no adjustment is available that ensures that like cases are being compared. ANCOVA-following weighting is more robust than simple ANCOVA, but when the groups remain substantially differentiated after weighting, the ANCOVA results remain suspect.[2]

Weighting can make the target and comparison groups more comparable but it also has the effect of reducing the effective sample size of the comparison group (Table 5.2) for testing program effects. For instance, although every OP program begins with a comparison group

---

[1] The effect size used here is defined as the difference between target and comparison group means divided by the standard deviation for the target group. We use only the target group standard deviation so that changes in effect size before and after weighting result only from reductions in group mean differences, not from changes in the variability due to weighting the comparison group.

[2] Tests for treatment effects were not adjusted for multiple comparisons across the multiple outcome variables or for multiple comparisons across programs. No adjustments were made because the outcomes were specified in advance and our interest is in a program's effect on each outcome, not on its overall effect; we wanted to preserve the Type I error rates for individual outcome rather than maintain the familywise error across outcomes.

Table 5.2
Comparison Group Effective Sample Sizes After Weighting and Associated Minimum Detectable Effect Size

Program	Effective Sample Size of the Comparison Group	Minimum Effect Size Detectable with Probability 80%
LTR		
A	61.5	0.515
B	103.0	0.358
C	41.6	0.578
STR		
D	86.6	0.377
E	114.0	0.341
F	22.1	0.646
G	74.7	0.397
OP		
H	126.0	0.335
I	132.0	0.341
J	109.0	0.391

NOTE: 80 percent power, two-tailed, alpha = .05.

consisting of at least 400 cases, after weighting, no OP comparison group has an effective sample size greater than 126, and one has a comparison group with an effective sample size of less than 21.[3] This variability in the size of weighted comparison groups has implications for the power of our analyses to detect significant treatment effect estimates. To highlight these limitations, Table 5.2 provides the minimum effect size that we would expect to be able to detect 80 percent of the time, assuming a two-tailed t-test with alpha = 0.05.

As Table 5.2 illustrates, for just 7 of the 11 programs the effective sample sizes are sufficiently large so that we could expect to have had about an 80 percent chance (power of .80) of detecting effect sizes between 0.2 and 0.4 (which are commonly considered small to medium effects, but which might be hard to achieve for relative treatment effects). Treatment effect estimates for three other programs would need to be in the range of .4 to .8 for our study to have had an 80 percent chance of detecting the relative treatment effects. Finally, the effective sample size for one program is so small that the true treatment effect would have to be equal to a whole standard deviation for us to have had an 80 percent chance of detecting it. Using covariate adjustment will reduce our power relative to the power for the weighted comparison of means. Thus, for several of the programs there is a sizeable probability that small effects or even moderate treatment effects cannot be detected because the samples are small and the programs are serving relatively distinct populations.

---

[3] In our analyses we treat the propensity score weights as fixed. This can overestimate standard errors because it ignores the reduction in variability in the estimated treatment effect that results from selecting weights that maintain balance. However, good estimates of standard errors with GBM-based propensity scores have not fully been established, and sample reuse methods were not feasible for this study. Hence we use this conservative approach. The power calculations are consistent with our conservative approach to estimating standard errors.

CHAPTER SIX

Outcomes

Treatment effects for each program are presented below for each of the five selected outcomes. As discussed earlier, these treatment effects represent the differential benefits 12 months after admission to the target program, versus other programs in the same level of care, for youths like those typically attending the target program. We display these differences graphically as effect sizes with confidence intervals. The effect size is the difference score divided by the standard deviation of the outcome for the target facility. This measure provides a standardized outcome metric with which to compare programs on an outcome and across outcomes.

For each program and outcome, figures contain three estimated treatment effects (three methods for measuring the difference between the treatment and comparison groups on the outcome) and confidence intervals for each estimate. Thus, estimates plotted above the line at an effect size of 0 indicate that the treatment program had higher scores on the outcome than the comparison group. Treatment effect estimates below 0 indicate that the treatment program had lower scores on the outcome than the comparison group. The left-most effect is the unadjusted effect—the raw mean difference between groups standardized by the treatment group standard error. The bars above and below the effect size indicate the 95 percent confidence intervals for the effect size estimates. When these bars cross the horizontal line indicating an effect size of zero, this means that the observed treatment effect is not statistically significantly different than 0. The next effect for each outcome is the weighted estimate with youths from the comparison facilities weighted by their odds of receiving treatment at the target facility. The final estimate for each outcome is the estimated treatment effect adjusted by weighting and linear adjustments for variables that remain different after weighting, that is, the weighted analysis of covariance estimate.[1]

---

[1] The recovery outcome is dichotomous and we conducted our covariate adjustment on the log-odds scale using propensity score weighted logistic regression with covariates. To present the adjusted effect size on the probability scale, we used the logistic regression model to estimate the probability of recovery for all youths from both the target and comparison facilities, first assuming every youth received treatment at the target facility and then assuming they received treatment at the comparison facilities. We calculated the differences in these estimated probabilities, the weighted average of which is the estimate of the adjusted treatment effect of recovery. The standard errors we estimated using the delta method (Efron and Tibshirani, 1993) and the covariance matrix of the estimated logistic regression coefficients.

Long-Term Residential Programs

We first study the effects of the three long-term residential facilities in the ATM sample.

Program A

Figure 6.1 provides treatment effect estimates for Program A. Without adjustment (circles) there are significant differences between this facility and other LTR facilities on substance use problems and emotional problems. For both outcomes, youths attending Program A appear to have worse outcomes than those attending other programs in the LTR level of care. No other unadjusted treatment effects are significantly different than zero.

Weighting does not alter the appearance that Program A is having negative effects on emotional and substance problems (squares). However it does lead to an additional, marginally significant effect for substance use frequency, suggesting that youths attending Program A are using more drugs 12 months later than those attending other LTR programs who are most similar to youths entering Program A. Moreover, the effect for illegal activities increases with weighting, although the effect is not quite significant.

Figure 6.1
Treatment Effect Sizes for Program A (Effect sizes and 95-percent confidence intervals for outcome differences between programs and their comparison groups, unadjusted [circles], weighted [squares], and with covariate adjustment [diamonds])

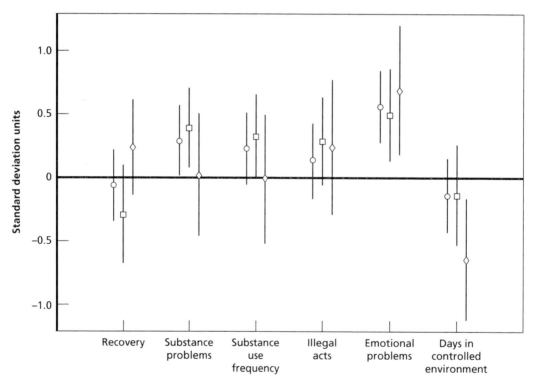

RAND TR346-6.1

As noted earlier, however, weighting failed to create a comparison group with covariate distributions sufficiently comparable to support strong treatment effect estimates. Table A.7 of the Appendix reveals that differences remain on measures of needle use, substance dependence, prior psychological treatment, mental health, and involvement with the criminal justice system among others. In particular, Program A cases have less needle use and lower substance dependence index scores than comparison LTR cases even after weighting. Without further adjustment we might confound these remaining differences with the causal effects of Program A. For example, if needle users tend to have worse outcomes regardless of the treatment program, we might overestimate the positive effects of Program A.

One additional adjustment we can make is to control for the effects of control variables that differ between the target and weighted comparison samples. This approach requires the assumption that even though groups are not very well matched, outcome differences are linearly associated with control variables on which they differ. We were able to reduce some of the distributional differences between the target and comparison groups, which makes the covariate adjustment more robust to violations of the linearity assumption. As planned, therefore, we produce a third estimate of the treatment effect using a weighted ANCOVA model that controls for all control variables with significant ($p < 0.05$) KS statistics after weighting. For Program A, 23 of the 86 control variables are selected using this criterion, so they were included in the ANCOVA estimate.

As Figure 6.1 illustrates, the ANCOVA models (diamonds) provide a different pattern of significant effects than either the weighted or unweighted estimates. Specifically, neither substance problems nor substance use frequency remain significant after ANCOVA adjustment, and the estimated effects are now essentially zero. However, the estimate for emotional problems is actually greater than earlier estimates and remains significant. In addition, detention is now significant, suggesting that those who attended Program A were less likely to be in a controlled environment 12 months later than comparable youths attending other LTR programs. This finding suggests one reason why substance problems and frequency, and criminal activity, may appear greater for Program A cases than their comparison cases: Program A may be better at keeping youths out of jail and in community settings where they remain at risk for drug use and other behavioral problems.

Program B

Having gone through the results for Program A in some detail, we present the remaining programs' results more cursorily. Figure 6.2 summarizes the results for Program B. Program B was one of the programs with a large and well-matched weighted comparison group. Therefore, we may be more interested in the weighted treatment effect estimates than in the ANCOVA treatment effects, since we expect no differences in the treatment effect estimates, but we expect the weighted analyses to provide estimates with smaller confidence intervals. In the case of Program B, however, there are no differences in the conclusions to be drawn from any of the three sets of treatment effect estimates. For every outcome there is no evidence, when considering only youths like those who typically attend Program B, that Program B provides an incremental advantage or disadvantage in 12-month outcomes.

Figure 6.2
Treatment Effect Sizes for Program B (Effect sizes and 95-percent confidence intervals for outcome differences between programs and their comparison groups, unadjusted [circles], weighted [squares], and with covariate adjustment [diamonds])

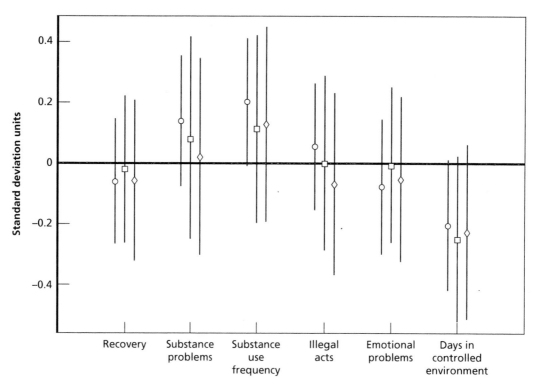

RAND *TR346-6.2*

Program C

Figure 6.3 suggests that there are extremely large outcome differences between youths attending Program C and those attending other LTR programs, even after weighting the comparison cases to look more like youths in Program C. Specifically, there are statistically significant treatment effects for this program for all outcomes except recovery in both the unweighted and weighted analyses. Indeed, estimates for the beneficial effect of Program C on substance problems range between 4 and 6 standard deviation units. Interestingly, ANCOVA adjustment has the effect of increasing, rather than diminishing, most of these already large treatment effects.[2] Overall, therefore, the results suggest that Program C is having strong beneficial effects on youths' substance problems, substance use frequency, illegal activities, and emotional problems. It is also associated with greater rates of detention 12 months later, which might help to explain one mechanism by which it is effecting the positive behavioral outcomes: With more youths in controlled environments, there is less opportunity to engage in drug use and other problem behaviors.

---

[2] The analysis of covariance model for recovery failed to converge due to instability with the dichotomous outcome and no results are reported.

Figure 6.3
Treatment Effect Sizes for Program C (Effect sizes and 95-percent confidence intervals for outcome differences between programs and their comparison groups, unadjusted [circles], weighted [squares], and with covariate adjustment [diamonds])

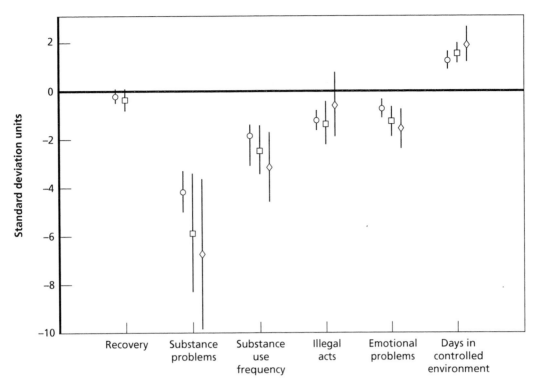

RAND *TR346-6.3*

Using auxiliary data we found that among Program C cases, nearly all the days in controlled environments were in treatment facilities rather than other institutions like jail or correctional centers. Eighty-eight percent of the cases from Program C report at least one day in a treatment facility and 76 percent report 90 days in a treatment facility in the 90 days preceding the 12-month follow-up interview. Only 3 percent of the Program C cases report any days in other controlled environments prior to the follow-up interview, and the maximum number of days is 4. For other LTR programs (including the comparison cases), only 19 percent of cases report any days in a treatment facility and only 7 percent report 90 days in such a facility. The data do not specify the source of treatment, but it is very clear that youths entering Program C and responding to the survey are much more likely to be receiving treatment 12 months later than are youths in other programs.

It must also be noted that Program C is the program with the least well-matched comparison sample (i.e., with the highest maximum KS statistic). In particular, cases in Program C have greater needle use and needle problems than the comparison cases, even after weighting. Given that youth with needle use and needle problems are typically considered difficult to treat, we might expect treatment effect estimates to be negatively biased.

Figure 6.4 summarizes the treatment effects for the residential programs. For each site the plot includes the adjusted estimate that we feel best controls for pretreatment differences. The adjusted estimates suggest that youths treated in Program C differ from youths in other facilities 12-months after treatment entry in terms of having fewer substance use problems, less frequent substance use, fewer emotional problems, and more days in a controlled environment. The only other significant effect is for youths receiving care in Program A who tend to have more emotional problems than we expect they would have, had they received care at one of the other sites.

Figure 6.4
Treatment Effect Sizes for Residential Facilities (Effect sizes and 95-percent confidence intervals for outcome differences between programs and their comparison groups)

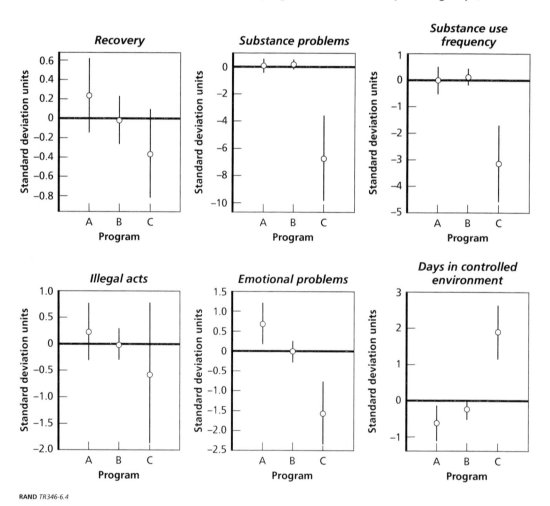

RAND TR346-6.4

Short-Term Residential Programs

Program D

Before weighting there are statistically significant differences between this facility and the comparison STR facilities only on emotional problems (Figure 6.5). The same pattern of results is observed after weighting. The ANCOVA adjusted outcomes, however, eliminate all significant differences. However, differences remain on several control variables between Program D and its weighted comparison cases. These variables include the needle frequency index, needle use, need for heroin treatment, and use of opiates, for which cases in Program D reported higher values than their counterparts in the other STR programs. Cases in Program D were also more likely to be in jail prior to treatment, less likely to be in school, had lower vocational risk, lower training activity, and low values on the high resistance measure than the weighted comparison cases. Because of the remaining difference on the pretreatment control variables between Program D and the weighted comparison group, the ANCOVA results probably represent the most reliable treatment effect estimates for this program.

Figure 6.5
Treatment Effect Sizes for Program D (Effect sizes and 95-percent confidence intervals for outcome differences between programs and their comparison groups, unadjusted [circles], weighted [squares], and with covariate adjustment [diamonds])

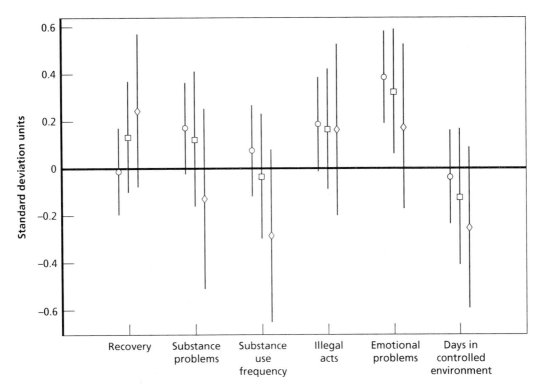

Program E

Program E tended to have higher values on criminal justice system indicators than the weighted comparison cases with higher values on the controlled environment index, the current criminal justice status, and the criminal justice system index. The cases in this program were also more likely to be Mexican than at other STR programs and reported greater use of cocaine.

Unweighted, weighted, and ANCOVA treatment effect estimates suggest that Program E is associated with significantly reduced chances of being in recovery at 12 months, and with reduced emotional problems (Figure 6.6). It also appears to be associated with increased rates of days CE in the unweighted and weighted analyses, but not in the ANCOVA model where the estimated difference is substantially smaller than the other two estimates. The increased levels of days CE for this program might be the source of the lower rate of recovery.

Figure 6.6
Treatment Effect Sizes for Program E (Effect Sizes and 95-percent confidence intervals for outcome differences between programs and their comparison groups, unadjusted [circles], weighted [squares], and with covariate adjustment [diamonds])

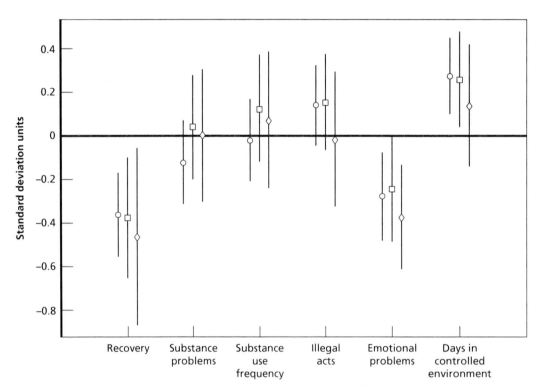

RAND *TR346-6.6*

Program F

Program F serves an especially unique population of clients, who differ on a number of pre-treatment covariates from those clients seen in every other ATM program. As a result, weighting fails to eliminate important pretreatment differences between Program F clients and the best available comparison sample of STR cases. Because of these substantial pretreatment differences, the unweighted outcome differences between Program F and all cases entering other STR programs is large and significant for all outcomes other than days CE (Figure 6.7). Weighting, however, eliminates all significant differences, and changed the direction of three treatment effects. Weighting greatly inflated the standard errors, because very few youths in the comparison group matched the population served by this program. Because differences remain on several pretreatment variables after weighting, the ANCOVA includes many covariates and the estimates become unstable as demonstrated by the large confidence intervals. Thus, even with our extensive case-mix adjustment, it is difficult to interpret the observed differences, and the data can provide only very limited information about the effects of this program.

Figure 6.7
Treatment Effect Sizes for Program F (Effect sizes and 95-percent confidence intervals for outcome differences between programs and their comparison groups, unadjusted [circles], weighted [squares], and with covariate adjustment [diamonds])

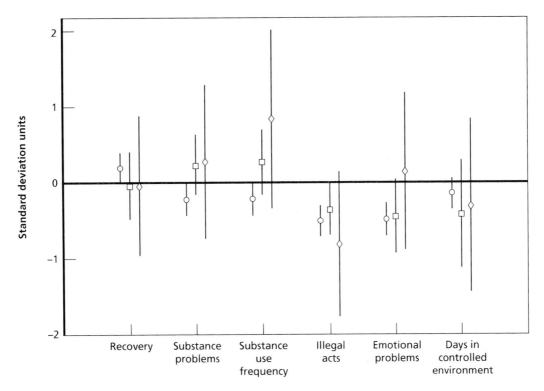

Program G

Prior to weighting there are significant differences between this program and other STR facilities on youths' emotional problems and days CE at 12 months following the intervention (Figure 6.8). The differences for emotional problems remain after weighting, but not after additional linear adjustments for covariates that remain different across groups after weighting. However, Program G is one of the sites for which a good weighted comparison group was identified; therefore, we focus on the weighted treatment effects, concluding that the only treatment effect on which Program G appears to differ from other STR programs is that of being associated with increased emotional problems 12 months after admission.

Figure 6.9 summarizes the results for STR facilities. Youths receiving care in Program E are less likely to be in recovery but have fewer emotional problems than had they received care at one of the other STR facilities. Otherwise there are no significant differences among the STR sites.

Figure 6.8
Treatment Effect Sizes for Program G (Effect sizes and 95-percent confidence intervals for outcome differences between programs and their comparison groups, unadjusted [circles], weighted [squares], and with covariate adjustment [diamonds])

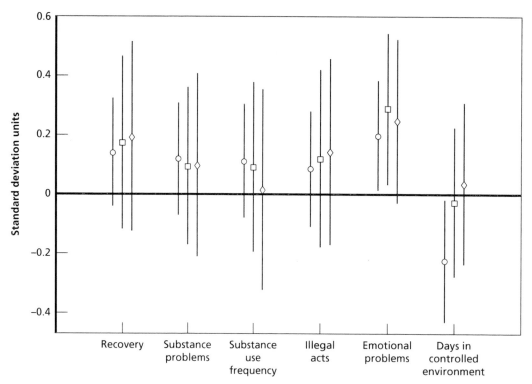

Figure 6.9
Treatment Effects for Short-Term Residential Facilities (Effect sizes and 95-percent confidence intervals for outcome differences between programs and their comparison groups)

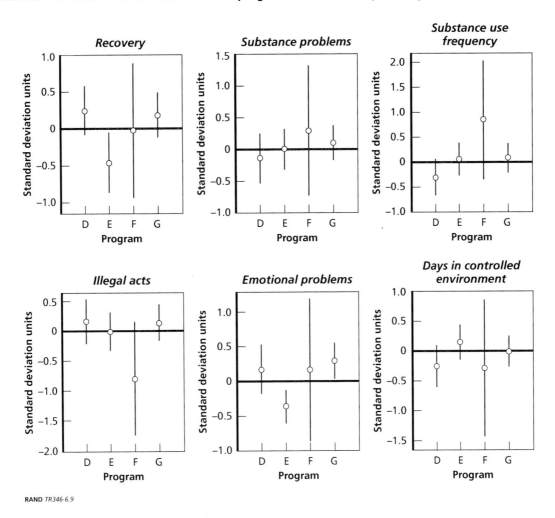

RAND *TR346-6.9*

Outpatient Programs

Program H

Prior to weighting, the outcomes of youths treated at Program H are worse for substance use frequency, illegal acts, and emotional problems, and better for days CE than youths treated in the other outpatient facilities (Figure 6.10). After adjusting for pretreatment differences through weighting, differences remain for both illegal acts and emotional problems. Adjusting for a small number of covariates including higher raters of need for heroin treatment than at the other OP facilities removes these remaining effects. Nevertheless, the weighted comparison group appears to have been a good one, in that differences in the distribution of control variables was within the range that would be expected in a random assignment study. Therefore, we conclude that treatment at Program H is, in fact, associated with worse criminal activity and emotional problems 12 months after admission.

Figure 6.10
Treatment Effect Sizes for Program H (Effect sizes and 95-percent confidence intervals for outcome differences between programs and their comparison groups, unadjusted [circles], weighted [squares], and with covariate adjustment [diamonds])

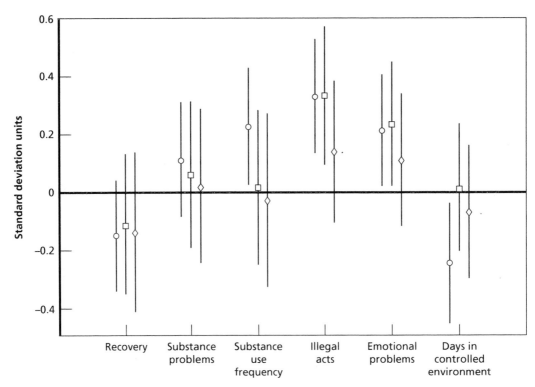

Program I

Prior to weighting the outcomes for youths treated in Program I, statistically significant effects are observed for recovery, illegal acts, and emotional problems (Figure 6.11). However, after adjusting for pretreatment differences through weighting, none of the differences are statistically significant. In most cases, the loss of statistical significance results from the slightly reduced precision of the weighted estimates, rather than from large changes in the estimated effects. Although the ANCOVA treatment effect estimates again reveal a significant detrimental effect of Program I on emotional problems, the weighted comparison group provided a good match to cases treated in Program I, raising questions about the need for ANCOVA adjustment.

Figure 6.11
Treatment Effect Sizes for Program I (Effect sizes and 95-percent confidence intervals for outcome differences between programs and their comparison groups, unadjusted [circles], weighted [squares], and with covariate adjustment [diamonds])

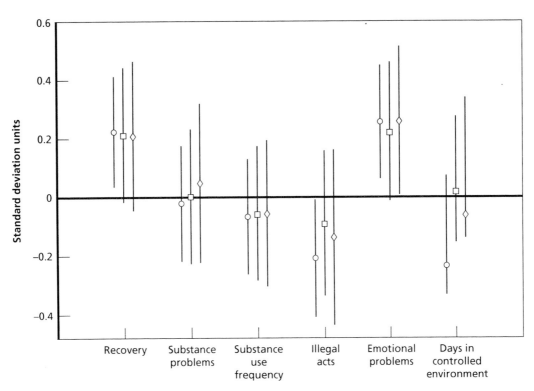

Program J

Regardless of the estimator, Site J appears to have reduced youths' emotional problems relative to the other outpatient facilities 12 months after program admission (Figure 6.12). Youths from this facility also have a higher level of days CE 12 months after intake, but that difference appears to be a result of pretreatment differences in the populations served by the facilities and it is not present after case-mix adjustment. Some caution in interpreting the results is probably warranted because youths from Program J had high values of substance dependence compared to the other OP programs even after weighting. Program J cases had higher values on the substance dependence index, substance abuse treatment index, the controlled environment index, and the current treatment index. They also had higher levels of methamphetamine use, victimization, withdrawal, prior opiate use, and time in treatment.

Figure 6.13 summarizes the treatment effect estimates for the outpatient facilities. Program H appears to perform less well at helping youths who receive care at this facility with curbing illegal activities or controlling emotional problems than the other outpatient facilities in the study. There are no other statistically significant effects and no patterns in the effect estimates exist.

Figure 6.12
Treatment Effect Sizes for Program J (Effect sizes and 95-percent confidence intervals for outcome differences between programs and their comparison groups, unadjusted [circles], weighted [squares], and with covariate adjustment [diamonds])

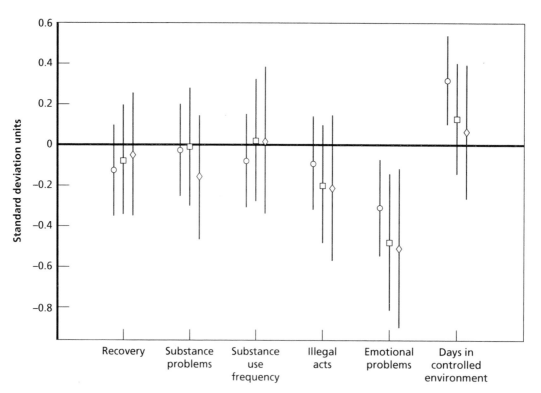

RAND *TR346-6.12*

Figure 6.13
Treatment Effects for Outpatient Facilities (Effect sizes and 95-percent confidence intervals for outcome differences between programs and their comparison groups)

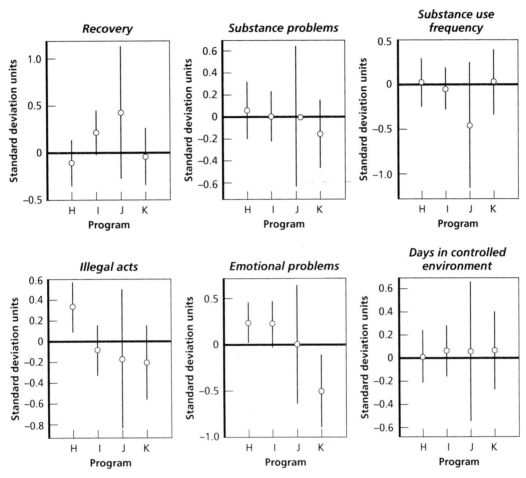

CHAPTER SEVEN

Discussion

Parents, purchasers, and other stakeholders have a strong interest in knowing which adolescent substance abuse treatment services are most effective at reducing substance use and other problems. Currently, however, no such information is available about the kinds of programs most commonly available to youths. Similarly, little is known about what might constitute "best practices" in the treatment of adolescent substance abusers. Thus, whereas in other areas of the healthcare system, quality of care and quality improvement over time is measured using indicators such as the proportion of cases receiving accepted standards of care (e.g., McGlynn et al., 2003), no such quality of care framework is yet available for adolescent substance abuse treatment.

Without process of care indicators, many have concluded that measurement of treatment program performance must be based on program outcomes. For instance, SAMHSA recently launched its State Outcomes Measurement and Management System (SOMMS), an outcomes monitoring program designed to facilitate evidence-based decisionmaking and quality improvement by establishing substance abuse treatment performance benchmarks (SAMHSA, July 2005). State outcome monitoring systems have previously been used to examine state-level trends in substance abuse treatment care. In contrast to this type of system description, which attempts to use outcome data to isolate differences in treatment performance across treatment programs, types of care, modalities, or geographic regions, must first overcome very challenging methodological obstacles. These include, for instance, the small number of cases available for review at any one program, client heterogeneity across programs, and differences across programs in rates of available outcome data, to name just a few.

In this report we explore the feasibility of using outcome data to evaluate adolescent drug treatment program performance, using the largest, most complete dataset available at the time we initiated this study, SAMHSA's ATM program dataset. Specifically, we explore the use of a causal modeling framework for establishing whether any ATM program appears to be more effective on a range of outcomes than any other in the same level of care.

Treatment effectiveness has often been gauged by comparing client severity before and after receiving treatment services. By this convention, all ATM programs were highly effective. For instance, every program was associated with significant reductions in drug use and drug problems. Clearly, however, these improvements conflate the treatment effects of interest (i.e., the effect of the treatment program) with the effects of normal maturation, regression to the mean, and other unwanted effects. Similarly, comparison of such changes tells us little about which programs are most effective, since those with the largest improvements may have treated clients that were substantially different, and perhaps more easy to treat, than those with smaller change scores.

We could establish one estimate of the relative effectiveness of different treatment programs by randomly assigning cases to each program, and then comparing their outcomes. This would ensure that any differences in outcomes would be attributable to the programs themselves, rather than to differences in the risk profiles of the clients they serve. This approach, however, assumes that every program should be able to treat every case. If programs specialize in caring for a particular type of adolescent, this approach might mask this program competency. If, for instance, a program designed for pregnant adolescent drug users does not work well for males, this should not be cited as evidence that it is ineffective for its target population.

We address these challenges by developing new case-mix adjustment techniques to compare 12-month outcomes of youths entering each program to the same outcomes for youths who attended another program in the same level of care, after weighting these cases to have covariate distributions comparable to the cases entering the target program. Thus, we consider the treatment effect expected for those who typically enter the program, rather than, for instance, the treatment effect that might be expected for any youth seeking treatment at any program. Furthermore, by ensuring that program outcomes are compared only with youths comparable to those treated at the program on 86 variables associated with ASAM placement criteria, we improve our chances of detecting true treatment effects, as opposed to outcome differences that result from pretreatment differences between treatment and comparison groups.

Assuming that the ASAM criteria do, in fact, describe important risk factors for later functioning, then one important finding in this report is that each of the programs is serving a group of youths with distinctly different risk profiles, suggesting that failure to account for these differences in comparisons of programs will produce biased conclusions. Before weighting there were large and significant differences between every target program and its corresponding comparison programs. These differences were often for clearly important risk factors such as pretreatment substance use and the use of needles and opiates. Weighting by the propensity scores removes many of these differences, but it did not eliminate all pretreatment group differences for some programs. In these cases, we used weighted ANCOVA methods in an attempt to control for the remaining group differences.

As summarized in Table 7.1, the effect of these adjustments was to eliminate most of the apparent treatment effects observed before case-mix adjustment. Across the 66 program and outcome pairings, only 11 statistically significant treatment effects were observed, and the target facility had a positive effect relative to the comparison facilities in only five of these pairs. In these pairs, adolescent outcomes following treatment in the target facility were better than those of comparable cases in the comparison facility. The remaining statistically significant effects were negative. That is, adolescent outcomes following treatment in the target facility were worse than those of comparable cases in the comparison facility, which does not imply that outcomes were worse than they would have been without treatment.

Table 7.1
Summary of Treatment Effect Estimates, Analysis Power, and Quality of Weighted Comparison Groups

	LTR			STR				OP		
Program	A	B	C	D	E	F	G	H	I	J
Outcome[a]										
Recovery	0.24	−0.02	−0.37	0.25	−0.46[d]	−0.03	0.18	−0.11	0.21	−0.05
Subst. probs	0.03	0.08	−6.71[d]	−0.13	0.01	0.29	0.10	0.06	0.00	−0.16
Subst. freq	−0.01	0.11	−3.16[d]	−0.29	0.07	0.85	0.09	0.02	−0.06	0.02
Illegal Acts	0.24	0.00	−0.57	0.17	−0.02	−0.80	0.12	0.34[d]	−0.09	−0.21
Emot. Probs	0.69[d]	−0.01	−1.56[d]	0.18	−0.37[d]	0.16	0.29[d]	0.24[d]	0.22	−0.51[d]
Cont. Env.	−0.64[d]	−0.25	1.90[d]	−0.25	0.14	−0.30	−0.03	0.02	0.06	0.07
Estimate Quality										
MDES[b]	0.52	0.36	0.58	0.38	0.34	0.65	0.40	0.34	0.34	0.39
Weights[c]	U	B	U	U	U	U	B	B	B	U

[a] Negative effect sizes indicate that outcomes at the treatment program are superior to those at comparison programs. Positive effect sizes indicate the treatment program had worse outcomes. For controlled environment, negative effect sizes indicate the treatment program had less controlled environment time at follow up than comparison sites. Positive effect sizes indicate the treatment program had more controlled environment time than the comparison group.

[b] MDES = Minimum detectable effect sizes for power of 0.8.

[c] When weighting results in a maximum KS statistic across 86 control variables that are as small or smaller than would be expected, in at least 10 percent of random assignment studies with the same variables, the estimate is denoted with a "B" for balanced. Otherwise, it is denoted with a "U" for unbalanced.

[d] Significant treatment effect estimate ($p < .05$).

The presence of six significant and negative effects is somewhat surprising given we are estimating each program's effect on its client population. However, the meaning of these negative effects is not altogether clear. First, half of these effects are for a single outcome variable, emotional problems. The relationship of this outcome to other traditional substance abuse treatment outcomes is ambiguous. It could be argued, for instance, that some emotional distress might be an expected correlate of abstinence from the substances previously used to medicate or avoid emotional problems. Similarly, a fourth apparently negative effect is the finding that Program C is associated with increased days in a controlled environment. However, Program C was planned as a 12-month treatment, and nearly all the controlled environment days described 12 months after admission were attributable to those youths who were still in the controlled environment of Program C itself. In the context of an LTR program designed to treat youths for a year or more, retaining youths in the treatment program for a longer duration than the other LTR programs may be seen as a beneficial effect. More difficult to explain is the negative effect of Program E on recovery, and of Program H on illegal activities, the latter of which also benefited from a particularly good case-mix adjusted comparison group.

Only Program C stands out as having consistently positive outcomes, but the apparent effectiveness of this program may well be misleading. Over 75 percent of the program's cases were in treatment the entire 90 days prior to the 12-month survey. As a result Program C appears to outperform other programs in terms of 12-month substance problems, substance use frequency, and emotional problems. Although the weighted comparison group constructed for Program C differed from the treatment group by more than would be expected had groups been formed by random assignment, the differences tended to place Program C cases at greater risk of poor outcomes than their weighted counterparts in the comparison sample. However, Program C was exceptional in that it lost to follow-up more than 25 percent of its sample at the 12-month interview, compared to the excellent overall average follow-up rater of 91 percent. This level of study attrition can result in outcomes biased toward better outcomes than would be observed with lower attrition (Scott, 2004). In particular, if youths who left treatment are harder to find at follow-up, the sample from Program C might be biased in favor of high treatment retention rates and good outcomes. However, even if the entire sample lost to follow-up were not in treatment, Program C would still have a positive effect on treatment retention relative to the comparison programs. Thus, even with the differential attrition rates it is clear that Program C had positive effects on treatment retention and possibly other outcomes as a result.

Why Do We Find Few Differential Treatment Benefits?

The surprising scarcity of detectable treatment effects may be attributable to a number of factors, and perhaps most importantly to the limited statistical power available in many of the outcome analyses. The large differences between program clients served at each of the sites resulted in small effective sample sizes for many of the weighted comparison groups. Combined with the small sample sizes in several programs, the result was limited power to detect the kinds of small or even medium-sized treatment effects that might be expected in examination of relative treatment effects. As noted in Table 7.1, many of the treatment effect analyses had relatively poor power to detect significant differences. Indeed, none of these analyses had customarily acceptable levels of power to detect effect sizes smaller than 0.30. Moreover, these power analyses only concern the comparisons of weighted outcome means. The weighted ANCOVA might have lower power. Thus, it is likely that any real program differences that are small would go undetected in this report.

As noted above, this report uses aggressive case-mix adjustments to avoid bias in estimated effects. Omitting control variables that are even weakly associated with the outcome can result in significant bias in the treatment effect estimates. However, the cost of such aggressive case mix can be a loss in power. Interestingly, in many cases described in this report, it is not clear that weighting and the consequent reduction in effective sample size was the limiting factor for power. As can be seen in most of the outcome figures, standard errors for the treatment effect estimates were approximately equal before and after weighting, suggesting that reductions in sample size were compensated for by improvements in estimate precision. Future analyses should seek to evaluate treatment effects using larger samples, or by improving power in other ways, for example, better designs with groups designed to be highly similar, such as that used by the Adolescent Outcomes Project (Morral, McCaffrey, and Ridgeway, 2004).

Limited statistical power does not explain, however, why so many of our outcome analyses revealed small point estimates of program treatment effects, especially on measures of substance use, substance use problems, and substance use frequency indices. This finding is interesting and surprising, particularly given the case-mix adjustment perspective we adopted for these analyses. This perspective was designed to detect treatment effects resulting from adaptations programs have made to the specific characteristics of the clients they typically serve. As such, the findings of this report are similar to those reported from the Cannabis Youth Treatment project (Dennis et al., 2004) and Project MATCH (Matching Alcoholism Treatment to Client Heterogeneity) (Project Match Research Group, 1997). Specifically, differential treatment effects are not found, even though programs are compared, in some cases, to interventions involving fairly minimal treatment.

One interpretation of the modest evidence of effectiveness found in this study may be that it is due to limitations of examining relative, rather than absolute treatment effects. That is, we compare outcomes associated with each program to those associated with other programs in the same level of care. As such, the treatment effects we estimate tell us how much better or worse each program is than other comparable programs. This kind of relative treatment effect is useful for consumers faced with a choice of sending youths with specific characteristics to one or another treatment program, but they tell us little about absolute treatment effects, or the difference between the outcomes expected for youths treated at a program versus not treated at all.

Relative treatment effects yield ambiguous results. For instance, our finding that no STR or OP program appears to be more effective than its comparison programs at reducing substance use or substance problems admits a number of interpretations.

- If all programs had poor absolute treatment effects on these outcomes, we might expect no relative treatment effects.
- If all programs had very large, but equivalent, absolute treatment effects, on these outcomes, we would similarly expect no relative treatment effects.
- If the comparison sample is drawn from some programs that are more effective and some that are less effective than the program being evaluated, we might expect to find no relative treatment effects.

Moreover, even if relative differences do exist, we might expect them to be smaller than the effects we would find when comparing treatment to a no-treatment alternative, and our analyses might have less power to detect relative differences than they would to detect difference against a control.

The possibility that all programs were effective, thereby reducing the chances of noting differential or relative treatment effects is worth considering. The 11 programs evaluated under ATM were not a random sample of community-based substance abuse treatment programs for adolescents. They were, in fact, selected by CSAT for evaluation because they were able to demonstrate some evidence of effectiveness. Thus, the range of outcomes these programs produced may well have been unusually good. Nevertheless, not all of the cases used as comparison cases for this study were drawn from the 11 potentially exemplary programs selected for evaluation under ATM. In both the LTR and OP levels of care, cases treated at other programs included in the ATM study to serve as comparison cases for local evaluations were available for inclusion in comparison groups reported in this analysis. More than half of the available comparison groups in each of the LTR analyses were treated at programs other than the three LTR programs evaluated under ATM. Between 28 percent and 39 percent of the OP comparison groups consisted of youths treated at non-ATM OP treatment programs. Thus, for both the LTR and OP analyses, we might not expect the outcomes to be uniformly good due to selection of only exemplary treatment programs. This would only be true, however, if the non-ATM programs were not comparably exemplary, something we cannot determine with certainty.

Finally, our failure to find strong and persuasive evidence of treatment effectiveness could indicate that we were looking for that evidence in the wrong place. Large and significant treatment effects might exist for each evaluated treatment program, but these might be no longer detectable 12 months after treatment admission. McLellan et al (2005) have argued, for instance, that for chronic, relapsing conditions like substance abuse, the treatment effects of interest are chiefly those observed during treatment. By analogy, they note that treatments for other chronic conditions, like diabetes or schizophrenia, are typically evaluated in terms of symptom management during treatment, not by whether or not such benefits remain detectable long after treatments are withdrawn.

Whereas this argument has considerable appeal for treatment of adult chronic substance abusers, the applicability to adolescent substance abusers, many of whom appear to be in the early stages of substance abuse, is not yet well established. Clearly parents and other stakeholders would like to identify treatments that have long-lasting effects, making the evaluation of 12-month outcomes for adolescent treatments a valid, if nevertheless unpromising, enterprise.

Limitations

As with all evaluations, there are limitations on the conclusions that may legitimately be drawn from the findings reported here. In this section, we discuss what we believe are the most important of these limitations.

Case-Mix Adjustment May Be Imperfect

Important unmeasured pretreatment characteristics could exist, which, if included in our case-mix adjustments, would affect the outcome analyses. Exclusion of any such "hidden variables" would result, therefore, in our outcome results being biased.

Our findings illustrate that *unadjusted* treatment effect estimates can be clearly and strongly biased. Program F, for instance, appeared to have significant and beneficial effects on nearly every outcome before adjustment. This proved to be entirely due to the unique characteristics of the youths it serves. Thus, after accounting for Program F's unusually low risk mix of cases, four of the treatment effects that previously suggested beneficial treatment effects reversed direction, revealing negative effects, although these were not significant.

Although inclusion of any currently hidden variables would further reduce this bias, we may be confident that our adjusted results present a picture of the relative program effects that is much closer to the true relative effects than is often exhibited in observational substance abuse treatment evaluation research.

Each of the case-mix adjustment analyses presented in this report adjusts for between-group differences on 86 pretreatment control variables that could bias treatment outcome comparisons. The strength of our approach is further enhanced by a number of innovations:

- The inclusion of many highly reliable scales available in the GAIN-I survey instrument.
- The inclusion of an unprecedented number and diversity of variables that might be associated with both treatment selection and treatment outcomes.
- The adjustment for pretreatment characteristics identified by ASAM as theoretically and empirically relevant to placement decisions.
- The use of data-adaptive, nonparametric regression techniques that substantially reduce the risk of model misspecification due to the strong assumptions imposed in more common linear regression approaches to case-mix adjustment (McCaffrey, Ridgeway, and Morral, 2004).
- The explicit demonstration of the effect of our case-mix adjustment weights on the pretreatment differences between each program and its comparison group on all pretreatment control variables (see Tables Appendix). In contrast, the vast majority of published studies using case-mix adjustment fail to report the effects of those techniques on pretreatment group differences.
- Relatedly, our evaluation of comparability of target and comparison covariate distributions not just at the mean (as is the case when T-tests are used to assess balance), but across the entire distribution, using the KS statistic.
- Our use of randomization tests to evaluate whether remaining differences between target program and comparison group covariate distributions are larger than would be expected had groups been formed by random assignment.
- The use of propensity score weighting as the principal source of case-mix adjustment. Propensity score weighting allows for case-mix adjustment to be conducted without reference to the effect of the model on outcomes. In comparison, analysis of covariance and other case-mix adjustment approaches that model outcomes require model development to occur on the outcomes being evaluated. This creates opportunities for confirmatory biases to influence model development decisions.
- The use of ANCOVA and weighting to adjust for variables that remain differentially distributed across target and comparison groups after weighting.

On the basis of these innovations, we are confident that this report describes an unusually rigorous case-mix adjustment effort.

Although the possibility of hidden bias represents a real study limitation, the likely effects of any such variables on our findings is probably small. We have succeeded in including pretreatment control variables that we have both theoretical and empirical reasons to believe are the most important predictors of outcomes. For instance, in preliminary analyses we confirmed that across hundreds of available predictors, the pretreatment values of each outcome measure proved to be the best predictors of the outcome value. Thus, all but one of the outcome measures' pretreatment values were included as control variables in the propensity score analyses, and as control variables in treatment effect analyses when the propensity scores failed to balance them sufficiently across groups (the baseline value of the dichotomous recovery variable was not included in these analyses, because it lacked variability prior to treatment). It strikes us as highly unlikely that any hidden variable would account for more of the variance in any outcome than this baseline measurement of the outcome. Indeed, a more reasonable estimate of the possible magnitude of hidden variable effects would probably be the second most important predictor of each outcome. In every case, however, these second-best predictors account for too little variance in the outcome to introduce much bias in our program evaluation results, if they had been omitted.

At Best, the Treatment Effects Described in This Report Are at the Level of the Service Delivery Unit, Rather Than the Intervention Level

Our approach calculates a single relative treatment effect estimate for each program, which necessarily obscures within-program variations in available treatment services. Since most ATM programs offered a variety of services or interventions tailored to each youth's specific treatment needs, this means that each program's estimated treatment effect is an average of the individual treatment effects found for cases receiving different kinds of interventions. Indeed, two ATM programs conducted random assignment experiments in which clients received alternative interventions (e.g., Liddle et al., 2004). Our analyses necessarily ignore, or average across, such within-program variations in treatment effectiveness. Instead, all youths treated within a service delivery unit make up the treated cohort whose outcomes are measured against those of the comparison cases.

Similarly, the programs might be particularly effective at treating subgroups of their clients either through targeted interventions or for other reasons, but we might be unlikely to detect such superior effects when observing the programs' average treatment effects. Given the sample sizes available for this study, such subgroup and interaction analyses are not feasible but should be considered in future studies.

At Worst, the Treatment Effects Estimated in This Report Confound Program Level Effects with the Effects of Other Community Services

Each of the programs evaluated under ATM served youths in a different catchment area, with different types and amounts of other services and support available to them. Presumably, these additional available community resources could have a substantial impact on youths' 12-month outcomes. For instance, a relatively weak treatment program could still treat youths with good 12-month outcomes if many of those youths access other truly helpful services available to them in their communities. Similarly, strong programs in communities presenting a high risk of failure to youths might find that their clients are performing relatively poorly 12 months after program admission.

Ideally, this confound would be addressed by finding comparison cases from the same community or from communities with similar risk and protective factors. This kind of adjustment was not possible in the present study. Thus, the results we present must be understood as the effects of the program and community resources combined.

Twelve Months After Treatment Entry, Youths Have Different Exposures to Treatment and Risk

By design, or by differential drop-out rates, youths entering each evaluated program received differing durations of treatment and exposures to aftercare. As such, 12 months after program entry, when outcomes are assessed, youths from different programs may have been at risk for abusing drugs or other problems for differing durations. Arguably programs should be compared on the basis of equivalent doses of treatment and lengths of follow-up after discharge. This approach would answer the question, "If a youth were to receive equivalent doses of treatment at each program, which would have a greater effect?" We adopt a different perspective, and one which we believe to be more representative of the problem faced by those making practical referral decisions. Our approach answers the question: "Would the expected 12-month outcomes of a particular youth be superior if referred to one program versus to the others?"

Days in Controlled Environments at Follow-Up Present Important Challenges to Treatment Effect Estimation

Being in a controlled environment at follow-up affects key outcomes like substance use, substance problems, and criminal behavior. This creates difficult challenges for treatment effect estimation. For instance, if one program increases the chances of youths being imprisoned 12 months after admission, this program may appear to have very positive treatment effects on substance use and crime. Because reductions in these problems are secondary to incarceration, it would be incorrect to view such results as evidence of a beneficial treatment effect. Similarly, LTR programs that are especially good at retaining youths in treatment may appear to have beneficial effects on substance use and crime, because substantial numbers of cases are still in the controlled environment of treatment at follow-up. In this case, it is less clear whether these positive effects should be included or excluded as evidence of the program's effectiveness.

Treatment outcome studies rarely address the possible confounds presented by time in controlled environments. Nevertheless, treatment and juvenile justice detention is so common for adolescent substance abusers that it cannot be ignored in treatment effectiveness research. Figure 3.1, for instance, demonstrates that a year after entering LTR programs, ATM youths spent an average of 40 to 78 of their most recent 90 days in a controlled environment. Similarly, youths in STR and OP programs averaged sufficient numbers of days in controlled environments at follow-up to substantially affect their substance use, crime, and other outcomes.

A number of partial solutions have been suggested for addressing the controlled-environment confound. Among these, some analysts have examined treatment effectiveness only for the subset of cases who are free in the community at follow-up. Others suggest adjusting outcomes to account for detention at follow-up, by including this variable as a covariate in an analysis of covariance, or using risk-adjusted outcomes such as problems per day free in the community. Yet another approach is to define outcomes like our recovery variable, which account for both a functional outcome and the youths' detention status. Unfortunately, each of these approaches has serious shortcomings. The first two approaches ignore the possibility that detention is, itself, a part of the treatment effect. Rate-adjusted outcomes can be hard to interpret, are not defined for cases detained all 90 days, and may inappropriately assume linear associations between detention and outcomes like drug use problems. Combining quite different outcomes into a single index, like our recovery measure, requires a theory of the outcomes' true relationship and creates difficulties with interpretation. For example, is ongoing detention in a treatment facility good or bad, and is there a way to create a single index such that a higher score unambiguously implies more desirable outcomes when some youths are in treatment, some are in prison, and some are free in the community with and without drug use?

In this report we have not resolved the confound presented by days in controlled environments. Instead, we use the crude recovery variable, noting when its interpretation is complicated, for instance when youths complying with their LTR treatment plan are counted as being "not in recovery." In addition, we highlight for every program treatment effects on detention status and note when significant detention effects may complicate other observed treatment effects.

Other Less Significant Concerns

The data used to establish pretreatment characteristics as well as outcomes are based on self-reports that are subject to a variety of well-known biases. In the case of the present study, however, these problems are unlikely to bias our findings of relative treatment effects, unless there was differential response bias by site. Since there were a number of procedural differences in data collection, study design, and personnel across sites, differential response bias is a possibility. For instance, some evaluation teams were more or less closely identified with the programs they were evaluating, possibly resulting in different interview demand characteristics. To the extent participants in programs were sensitive to this factor and biased their responses accordingly, treatment effect estimates will be biased. We suspect, however, that any such confounded effects are probably small in magnitude if they exist at all.

No treatment program evaluation can provide conclusive evidence favoring one treatment approach over another. Even evaluations using the most rigorous study designs, involving the random assignment of cases to programs, cannot ensure that any observed differences in outcomes between conditions result from differences in the treatment approach (the factor intentionally manipulated in the study) rather than from a host of nonspecific factors over which experimental control is never complete in real-world studies, such as differences in programs' staff, resources, and physical environments.

Instead, conclusions about the relative efficacy of different treatment approaches should be based on an accumulation of rigorous evidence collected over multiple programs, different time periods, and, ideally, across multiple programs designed to implement each specific approach.

The analyses reported here represent a set of findings that should contribute to this accumulation of evidence.

Recommendations

In the absence of widely accepted and suitably specific quality-of-care indicators for adolescent substance abuse treatment, SAMHSA and many states are now exploring the use of outcomes-based performance measurement systems. The results from this study highlight a number of challenges to this plan and suggest strategies that should be considered in these and other efforts to understand treatment effects among individual programs, types of programs, or geographic regions.

1. Case-Mix Adjustment Is Important

The risk profiles of clients at different programs are quite variable. As a result, especially good or bad client outcomes may not reflect the performance of the treatment program, so much as the risk profiles of the clients it serves. Until the outcomes of comparable youths are compared, the relative effectiveness of different programs or groups of programs cannot be established. Similarly, if a program's client population changes over time, then comparisons of outcomes over time may not correspond to changes in that program's effectiveness. Finally, if risk profiles of clients differ by state, then comparisons of state treatment outcomes that fail to properly adjust for these differences are likely to be misleading.

2. Case-Mix Adjustment Is Not Enough

Even if the risk profiles of youths entering different programs were identical, this report highlights several ways in which valid conclusions about the effectiveness of different treatment programs may be difficult to draw from outcomes data. For instance, problems for interpretation arise when the proportion of cases providing follow-up data differs across programs. Thus, among the ATM programs, one had substantially lower rates of follow-up than the others, but the outcomes that were observed for this program appeared to be especially good. If those who are not followed up differed systematically from those who are, the outcomes for this program may be substantially more biased than those for the other ATM programs. Moreover, these are biases that may well be uncorrectable through, for instance, attrition weights, since the factors leading to study attrition may concern influences that occur long after the baseline assessment, such as nonresponsiveness to treatment. This suggests the need to ensure uniformly high rates of outcomes collection across programs.

Another challenge to the interpretation of outcomes concerns the high rates of institutionalization at follow-up observed in the ATM sample. When large proportions of cases are in controlled environments, many of the most important substance abuse treatment outcome measures are difficult to interpret. Thus, for instance, low levels of crime, drug use, and drug problems would ordinarily be viewed as a good outcome, but not if they reflect high rates of incarceration for a program's clients. Moreover, if programs from different geographic regions are compared, then differences in institutionalization rates cannot necessarily be attributed to treatment program effects. Instead, they might reflect differences in regional laws or law enforcement, the availability of inpatient services, or other community differences.

Indeed, community differences in resources, available support, opportunities, drug problems, and other characteristics may all influence the outcomes of youths in those communities, creating a significant confound for trying to establish effects specific to treatment programs on the basis of client outcomes, when those programs exist in different communities.

Each of these considerations suggest that even if case-mix adjustment is planned for outcomes-based performance measurement, valid conclusions about program performance may not be derivable from large-scale outcomes monitoring systems.

3. Program Differences May Be Small

In this report, no program was found to consistently outperform any other, across outcomes. Indeed, few program differences were noted on any outcome, even though 70 percent of these analyses had sufficient power to detect effect sizes of 0.40 or greater. If differences in program effectiveness are generally small, this means that in order to detect performance differences, the outcomes of larger numbers of cases must be assessed before sufficient data is available to draw desired inferences. Since some programs see only small numbers of cases, and since the collection of outcomes data is often expensive, this finding has important implications for the feasibility of using outcomes to assess differences in the performance of individual programs.

4. Outcomes-Based Performance Measurement May Be Impractical

Many of the challenges described above raise important questions about the feasibility of producing valid treatment performance information from large-scale outcome-based performance measurement efforts. This suggests that a more fruitful approach to performance measurement might be to invest more effort into identifying quality of care indicators for adolescent substance abuse treatment programs.

Supporting Tables

Table A.1
Summary of Means and Standard Deviations on All Baseline Control Variables by Program: Long-Term Residential

	Site A		Site B		Site C	
Variable	Mean	SD	Mean	SD	Mean	SD
Age	15.825	1.157	15.664	0.924	17.685	2.348
Times received treatment for drug/alc	0.930	1.269	4.362	16.617	1.963	4.207
Prior treatment psychological problems	0.684	0.465	0.191	0.393	0.352	0.478
No. people lived with[a]	7.053	12.959	4.704	8.529	4.352	5.303
Substance Dependence Index[a]	4.649	1.782	3.868	2.111	5.426	1.978
Substance Dependence Index[b]	0.877	1.523	1.730	2.167	2.944	2.738
Drug Crime Index, minus L3t	1.158	0.874	0.711	0.740	1.167	0.898
Living Risk Index	9.702	4.417	6.546	2.860	7.741	4.222
Vocational Risk Index	12.561	6.070	10.270	6.442	9.981	7.340
Social Risk Index	15.035	4.242	12.704	4.969	13.722	6.305
Needle Frequency Index	0.019	0.056	0.081	0.099	0.096	0.208
Needle Problem Index	0.281	1.484	0.184	1.085	1.389	2.965
Sex Protection Ratio	0.792	0.337	0.791	0.349	0.716	0.393
Controlled Environment Index	0.733	0.343	0.183	0.302	0.290	0.366
General Satisfaction Index	13.088	3.922	13.257	4.355	11.352	5.327
Mental Health Treatment Index	0.029	0.069	0.005	0.026	0.002	0.018
Criminal Justice System Index	0.843	0.330	0.539	0.482	0.303	0.426
Training Problem Index	5.158	1.833	5.408	2.014	3.389	3.246
Substance Abuse Treatment Index	0.048	0.133	0.045	0.138	0.094	0.211
Substance Problem Index[a]	11.474	3.283	9.618	3.789	12.167	4.017
Substance Problem Index[b]	2.649	3.814	4.500	4.614	6.796	5.746
Physical Health Treatment Index	0.021	0.031	0.017	0.035	0.027	0.061

Table A.1—Continued

Variable	Site A		Site B		Site C	
	Mean	SD	Mean	SD	Mean	SD
Internal Mental Distress Index	14.702	9.073	10.612	7.821	16.630	8.738
Environmental Risk Index	37.298	10.273	29.480	10.244	31.222	13.359
General Victimization Index	4.930	3.717	4.322	1.908	5.833	3.259
Personal Sources of Stress Index	2.456	1.511	1.461	1.366	2.333	1.478
Other Sources of Stress Index	2.614	1.890	1.612	1.747	2.204	1.747
Employment Problem Index	1.053	1.771	0.362	0.963	1.667	2.064
Employment Activity Index	0.155	0.277	0.166	0.297	0.211	0.344
Crime Violence Index	11.825	6.652	8.230	5.679	12.370	7.319
Illegal Activities Index	0.105	0.036	0.088	0.050	0.099	0.054
Substance Frequency Index	0.175	0.136	0.248	0.177	0.378	0.233
Current Withdrawal Index	1.158	3.211	1.941	3.917	5.852	6.355
Treatment Resistance Index	1.439	1.060	1.092	0.996	1.815	1.218
Treatment Motivation Index	3.228	0.991	2.625	1.245	3.185	0.883
Self-Efficacy Index	3.368	1.783	3.763	1.422	2.833	1.853
Problem Orientation Index	2.544	1.938	1.493	1.936	2.500	2.158
Health Problem Index	0.181	0.159	0.127	0.138	0.148	0.215
Behavior Complexity Index	16.965	6.572	12.414	7.359	17.685	8.027
Emotional Problem Index	0.342	0.238	0.248	0.171	0.338	0.218
General Social Support Index	7.211	1.745	6.520	1.987	6.185	2.195
Training Activity Index	0.649	0.212	0.558	0.301	0.247	0.300
Recovery Environment Risk Index	0.324	0.106	0.320	0.099	0.351	0.103
Prior opiate use	0.351	0.477	0.184	0.388	0.537	0.499
Need for heroin treatment (self-reported)	0.000	0.000	0.020	0.139	0.222	0.416
Seizures/current withdrawal symptoms	0.035	0.184	0.072	0.259	0.241	0.428
Using daily	0.579	0.494	0.836	0.371	0.852	0.355
Using opioids[d]	0.263	0.440	0.171	0.377	0.519	0.500
Used in past two days	0.018	0.131	0.013	0.114	0.093	0.290
Substance use despite prior treatment	0.088	0.283	0.099	0.298	0.204	0.403
Acute health problems	0.404	0.491	0.382	0.486	0.278	0.448
High behavioral problems[a]	0.474	0.499	0.197	0.398	0.574	0.494
Days of victimization[c]	0.175	0.380	0.283	0.450	0.259	0.438
High victimization	0.596	0.491	0.553	0.497	0.759	0.428
Current criminal justice involvement	0.930	0.255	1.000	0.000	0.759	0.428
Total arrests[c]	1.246	1.442	0.691	1.137	0.407	0.828
Mental distress	0.491	0.500	0.243	0.429	0.556	0.497
High resistance	0.158	0.365	0.099	0.298	0.296	0.457
Low motivation	0.211	0.408	0.382	0.486	0.204	0.403
Low alc/drug use problem orientation	0.298	0.457	0.566	0.496	0.407	0.491
First high/intoxicated under age 15	0.965	0.184	0.901	0.298	0.833	0.373
Needle use[c]	0.070	0.255	0.401	0.490	0.204	0.403
In school	0.965	0.184	0.829	0.377	0.463	0.499
Employed	0.246	0.430	0.243	0.429	0.278	0.448

Table A.1—Continued

Variable	Site A		Site B		Site C	
	Mean	SD	Mean	SD	Mean	SD
Homeless/runaway[a]	0.351	0.477	0.217	0.412	0.185	0.388
Family hist. of substance use	0.912	0.283	0.783	0.412	0.759	0.428
Weekly family problems[c]	0.386	0.487	0.474	0.499	0.574	0.494
Tobacco Dependence Index[b,c]	29.947	29.722	44.138	39.985	83.333	21.599
Health Distress Index[a]	2.158	1.056	1.888	1.104	2.204	1.177
Homicidal-Suicidal Thought Index	0.175	0.380	0.151	0.358	0.296	0.457
Lifetime detox admissions	0.018	0.131	0.270	0.803	1.278	3.679
Attended AA or other self-help	0.772	0.420	0.493	0.500	0.426	0.494
Last grade completed in school	8.947	1.317	8.967	1.274	9.481	1.675
Mention of alc as treatment need	0.404	0.491	0.059	0.236	0.241	0.428
Mention of marijuana as treatment need	0.596	0.491	0.342	0.474	0.519	0.500
Mention of cocaine as treatment need	0.053	0.223	0.158	0.365	0.296	0.457
Mention of opiates as treatment need	0.000	0.000	0.020	0.139	0.222	0.416
Mention of amph's as treatment need	0.246	0.430	0.178	0.382	0.019	0.135
Mention of other drugs as treatment need	0.123	0.328	0.013	0.114	0.148	0.355
Controlled environment[c]	45.632	27.759	15.809	25.889	21.148	29.443
Currently in alc/drug treatment	0.281	0.449	0.191	0.393	0.222	0.416
Gender						
Male	0.649	0.477	0.829	0.377	0.722	0.448
Female	0.351	0.477	0.171	0.377	0.278	0.448
Race						
Am. Indian	0.000	0.000	0.033	0.178	0.019	0.135
Black	0.228	0.420	0.079	0.270	0.148	0.355
White	0.439	0.496	0.204	0.403	0.352	0.478
Mexican	0.105	0.307	0.454	0.498	0.000	0.000
Other race	0.228	0.420	0.230	0.421	0.481	0.500
Substance most likes						
Alcohol	0.211	0.408	0.092	0.289	0.093	0.290
Cannabis	0.544	0.498	0.605	0.489	0.481	0.500
Crack or cocaine	0.035	0.184	0.125	0.331	0.130	0.336
Opiates	0.000	0.000	0.013	0.114	0.222	0.416
Hallucinogens	0.035	0.184	0.020	0.139	0.056	0.229
Amphetamines	0.158	0.365	0.132	0.338	0.019	0.135
Other substance	0.018	0.131	0.013	0.114	0.000	0.000
Current living status						
House/apt	0.544	0.498	0.750	0.433	0.778	0.416
Friend/relative	0.175	0.380	0.125	0.331	0.056	0.229
Jail/correctional	0.105	0.307	0.079	0.270	0.093	0.290
Other status	0.175	0.380	0.046	0.210	0.074	0.262

[a] Past year. [b] Past month. [c] Past 90 days. [d] Weekly.

Table A.2
Summary of Means and Standard Deviations on All Baseline Control Variables by Program: Short-Term Residential

Variables	Site D		Site E		Site F		Site G	
	Mean	SD	Mean	SD	Mean	SD	Mean	SD
Age	16.582	1.365	15.747	1.016	16.103	1.326	16.007	1.196
Times received treatment for drug/alc	2.190	2.622	1.145	3.904	1.159	2.037	1.114	2.224
Prior treatment psychological problems	0.562	0.496	0.337	0.473	0.214	0.410	0.678	0.467
No. people lived with[a]	4.444	3.483	4.783	4.845	4.762	2.287	4.054	2.717
Substance Dependence Index[a]	5.301	1.768	4.711	2.065	4.659	2.124	4.866	1.823
Substance Dependence Index[b]	3.039	2.703	1.843	2.260	1.611	1.894	3.356	2.241
Drug Crime Index, minus L3t	1.320	0.883	1.361	0.879	0.579	0.820	1.040	0.842
Living Risk Index	7.693	3.547	8.946	3.811	7.405	2.711	7.919	3.011
Vocational Risk Index	8.549	6.782	13.108	5.625	9.849	4.682	12.289	5.005
Social Risk Index	14.092	4.839	14.892	4.726	11.563	4.425	13.517	4.353
Needle Frequency Index	0.109	0.224	0.008	0.046	0.005	0.025	0.005	0.032
Needle Problem Index	1.503	2.964	0.084	0.605	0.071	0.645	0.161	0.997
Sex Protection Ratio	0.633	0.406	0.729	0.391	0.880	0.294	0.762	0.382
Controlled Environment Index	0.356	0.371	0.449	0.392	0.265	0.392	0.110	0.220
General Satisfaction Index	13.928	4.803	14.271	4.326	16.270	4.103	13.430	4.110
Mental Health Treatment Index	0.022	0.068	0.007	0.027	0.002	0.011	0.042	0.075
Criminal Justice System Index	0.622	0.446	0.798	0.381	0.525	0.477	0.236	0.398
Training Problem Index	3.680	2.738	4.614	2.346	3.992	2.177	5.201	1.810
Substance Abuse Treatment Index	0.066	0.128	0.038	0.109	0.089	0.199	0.085	0.183
Substance Problem Index[a]	12.163	3.419	11.651	3.550	10.857	3.806	11.201	3.464
Substance Problem Index[b]	7.118	5.707	5.012	4.810	4.000	3.895	8.154	4.310
Physical Health Treatment Index	0.016	0.040	0.018	0.036	0.006	0.012	0.016	0.019
Internal Mental Distress Index	12.366	9.131	15.048	8.786	10.603	8.905	14.020	8.308
Environmental Risk Index	30.333	10.303	37.024	8.727	28.810	8.559	33.725	8.854
General Victimization Index	5.020	3.107	6.175	3.420	4.310	2.991	5.087	2.956
Personal Sources of Stress Index	1.765	1.450	1.789	1.383	1.452	1.355	2.262	1.485
Other Sources of Stress Index	1.431	1.672	1.572	1.622	0.992	1.411	2.007	1.582
Employment Problem Index	2.268	2.117	1.325	1.798	0.714	1.327	1.262	1.743
Employment Activity Index	0.355	0.361	0.264	0.335	0.147	0.292	0.268	0.330

Table A.2—Continued

Variables	Site D Mean	Site D SD	Site E Mean	Site E SD	Site F Mean	Site F SD	Site G Mean	Site G SD
Crime Violence Index	13.039	6.722	12.355	6.153	6.111	5.451	10.430	5.427
Illegal Activities Index	0.115	0.052	0.107	0.044	0.068	0.053	0.115	0.050
Substance Frequency Index	0.367	0.187	0.247	0.162	0.145	0.147	0.318	0.169
Current Withdrawal Index	3.882	5.808	2.500	4.398	4.548	5.202	4.188	4.970
Treatment Resistance Index	1.379	1.010	1.518	1.057	1.730	1.034	1.966	1.089
Treatment Motivation Index	2.948	1.065	2.753	1.148	3.056	0.839	2.893	1.243
Self-Efficacy Index	3.739	1.366	3.584	1.537	3.563	1.428	3.409	1.589
Problem Orientation Index	2.444	2.099	2.217	1.976	2.024	1.974	2.591	1.997
Health Problem Index	0.146	0.177	0.179	0.163	0.054	0.091	0.181	0.136
Behavior Complexity Index	17.118	7.820	16.554	7.035	12.159	8.459	16.544	6.198
Emotional Problem Index	0.409	0.225	0.295	0.185	0.196	0.168	0.343	0.197
General Social Support Index	6.902	2.009	7.319	1.704	5.794	2.136	7.027	1.857
Training Activity Index	0.313	0.328	0.475	0.319	0.432	0.371	0.591	0.215
Recovery Environment Risk Index	0.334	0.097	0.363	0.115	0.240	0.072	0.385	0.106
Prior opiate use	0.536	0.499	0.343	0.475	0.135	0.342	0.470	0.499
Need for heroin treatment (self-reported)	0.294	0.456	0.006	0.077	0.008	0.089	0.000	0.000
Seizures/current withdrawal symptoms	0.183	0.387	0.145	0.352	0.206	0.405	0.195	0.396
Using daily	0.869	0.337	0.765	0.424	0.611	0.487	0.906	0.292
Using opioids[d]	0.392	0.488	0.367	0.482	0.016	0.125	0.336	0.472
Used in past two days	0.301	0.459	0.133	0.339	0.079	0.270	0.195	0.396
Substance use despite prior treatment	0.366	0.482	0.114	0.318	0.262	0.440	0.423	0.494
Acute health problems	0.346	0.476	0.446	0.497	0.135	0.342	0.497	0.500
High behavioral problems[a]	0.497	0.500	0.428	0.495	0.310	0.462	0.383	0.486
Days of victimization[c]	0.379	0.485	0.355	0.479	0.198	0.399	0.517	0.500
High victimization	0.745	0.436	0.747	0.435	0.667	0.471	0.752	0.432
Current criminal justice involvement	0.817	0.387	0.904	0.295	0.778	0.416	0.456	0.498
Total arrests[c]	0.843	0.997	0.928	1.382	0.937	2.666	0.557	1.071
Mental distress	0.627	0.483	0.452	0.498	0.286	0.452	0.436	0.496
High resistance	0.111	0.314	0.175	0.380	0.238	0.426	0.315	0.465
Low motivation	0.333	0.471	0.373	0.484	0.246	0.431	0.356	0.479
Low alc/drug use problem orientation	0.386	0.487	0.410	0.492	0.460	0.498	0.329	0.470
First high/intoxicated under age 15	0.869	0.337	0.964	0.187	0.897	0.304	0.926	0.261
Needle use[c]	0.209	0.407	0.024	0.153	0.016	0.125	0.013	0.115
In school	0.542	0.498	0.729	0.445	0.619	0.486	0.933	0.250

Table A.2—Continued

Variables	Site D Mean	Site D SD	Site E Mean	Site E SD	Site F Mean	Site F SD	Site G Mean	Site G SD
Employed	0.503	0.500	0.380	0.485	0.214	0.410	0.403	0.490
Homeless/runaway[a]	0.275	0.446	0.241	0.428	0.127	0.333	0.262	0.440
Family hist. of substance use	0.824	0.381	0.928	0.259	0.897	0.304	0.933	0.250
Weekly family problems[c]	0.477	0.499	0.518	0.500	0.159	0.365	0.651	0.477
Drunk/high most of day[d]	45.641	27.683	33.259	28.562	14.095	20.763	40.268	30.416
Tobacco Dependence Index[b,e]	67.974	27.964	48.584	34.121	27.238	31.469	59.846	35.618
Health Distress Index[a]	2.026	1.143	1.873	1.120	1.905	1.087	1.953	1.038
Homicidal-Suicidal Thought Index	0.183	0.387	0.241	0.428	0.238	0.426	0.396	0.489
Lifetime detox admissions	0.575	1.528	0.163	0.894	0.254	0.796	0.054	0.225
Attended AA or other self-help	0.588	0.492	0.367	0.482	0.508	0.500	0.530	0.499
Last grade completed in school	9.294	1.459	8.578	1.189	9.063	1.320	9.470	1.162
Mention of alc as treatment need	0.255	0.436	0.241	0.428	0.635	0.481	0.302	0.459
Mention of marijuana as treatment need	0.601	0.490	0.584	0.493	0.683	0.465	0.544	0.498
Mention of cocaine as treatment need	0.150	0.357	0.199	0.399	0.008	0.089	0.040	0.197
Mention of opiates as treatment need	0.320	0.467	0.006	0.077	0.008	0.089	0.000	0.000
Mention of amph's as treatment need	0.000	0.000	0.127	0.332	0.016	0.125	0.174	0.380
Mention of other drugs as treatment need	0.052	0.223	0.120	0.326	0.008	0.089	0.074	0.261
Controlled environment[c]	19.144	20.682	26.783	26.900	18.151	28.759	6.141	12.821
Currently in alc/drug treatment	0.157	0.364	0.193	0.394	0.127	0.333	0.262	0.440
Gender								
Male	0.784	0.411	0.699	0.459	0.651	0.477	0.638	0.481
Female	0.216	0.411	0.301	0.459	0.349	0.477	0.362	0.481
Race								
Am. Indian	0.020	0.139	0.012	0.109	0.944	0.229	0.027	0.162
Black	0.281	0.450	0.012	0.109	0.000	0.000	0.020	0.140
White	0.654	0.476	0.392	0.488	0.000	0.000	0.658	0.474
Mexican	0.000	0.000	0.404	0.491	0.000	0.000	0.067	0.250
Other race	0.046	0.209	0.181	0.385	0.056	0.229	0.228	0.420
Substance most likes								
Alcohol	0.105	0.306	0.096	0.295	0.214	0.410	0.208	0.406
Cannabis	0.569	0.495	0.651	0.477	0.770	0.421	0.664	0.472
Crack or cocaine	0.033	0.178	0.102	0.303	0.000	0.000	0.007	0.082
Opiates	0.235	0.424	0.006	0.077	0.000	0.000	0.000	0.000
Hallucinogens	0.052	0.223	0.054	0.226	0.000	0.000	0.020	0.140
Amphetamines	0.000	0.000	0.072	0.259	0.016	0.125	0.101	0.301
Other substance	0.007	0.081	0.018	0.133	0.000	0.000	0.000	0.000

Table A.2—Continued

Variables	Site D		Site E		Site F		Site G	
	Mean	SD	Mean	SD	Mean	SD	Mean	SD
Current living status								
House/apt	0.536	0.499	0.867	0.339	0.683	0.465	0.866	0.341
Friend/relative	0.078	0.269	0.066	0.249	0.048	0.213	0.101	0.301
Jail/correctional	0.314	0.464	0.006	0.077	0.032	0.175	0.007	0.082
Other status	0.072	0.258	0.060	0.238	0.238	0.426	0.027	0.162

[a] Past year.

[b] Past month.

[c] Past 90 days.

[d] Weekly.

Table A.3
Summary of Means and Standard Deviations on All Baseline Control Variables by Program: Outpatient Summary

Variables	Site H		Site I		Site J	
	Mean	SD	Mean	SD	Mean	SD
Age	15.955	1.067	15.906	1.154	15.557	1.045
Times received treatment for drug/alc	0.675	1.196	0.449	0.835	1.464	1.905
Prior treatment psychological problems	0.389	0.487	0.551	0.497	0.495	0.500
No. people lived with[a]	4.720	5.482	3.739	2.317	3.464	2.355
Substance Dependence Index[a]	2.478	2.071	2.949	2.198	4.598	2.123
Substance Dependence Index[b]	0.892	1.394	1.007	1.666	1.412	2.014
Drug Crime Index, minus L3t	0.701	0.709	0.551	0.713	0.866	0.892
Living Risk Index	7.070	2.952	6.406	2.786	7.546	3.840
Vocational Risk Index	8.662	5.301	9.580	4.256	10.155	6.126
Social Risk Index	11.229	4.975	10.246	3.755	12.423	5.700
Needle Frequency Index	0.007	0.055	0.002	0.015	0.009	0.059
Needle Problem Index	0.127	0.942	0.058	0.478	0.103	0.739
Sex Protection Ratio	0.813	0.349	0.817	0.347	0.763	0.403
Controlled Environment Index	0.154	0.328	0.169	0.311	0.396	0.374
General Satisfaction Index	16.331	4.408	15.855	3.941	13.598	5.076
Mental Health Treatment Index	0.011	0.074	0.010	0.029	0.026	0.110
Criminal Justice System Index	0.448	0.447	0.349	0.459	0.864	0.319
Training Problem Index	4.834	2.282	4.370	2.134	5.165	1.941
Substance Abuse Treatment Index	0.020	0.089	0.054	0.168	0.094	0.203
Substance Problem Index[a]	6.656	4.028	7.841	4.155	10.856	3.861
Substance Problem Index[b]	2.752	3.065	3.254	3.734	3.845	4.282
Physical Health Treatment Index	0.018	0.079	0.015	0.031	0.009	0.013
Internal Mental Distress Index	5.350	6.977	8.145	8.013	10.918	8.524
Environmental Risk Index	26.898	8.976	26.217	8.111	30.031	10.829
General Victimization Index	3.541	2.770	3.254	3.067	5.546	3.590

Table A.3—Continued

Variables	Site H		Site I		Site J	
	Mean	SD	Mean	SD	Mean	SD
Personal Sources of Stress Index	1.153	1.232	1.355	1.323	1.505	1.317
Other Sources of Stress Index	0.771	1.156	1.319	1.404	1.691	1.796
Employment Problem Index	1.535	1.602	1.500	1.612	1.052	1.410
Employment Activity Index	0.411	0.359	0.430	0.337	0.257	0.340
Crime Violence Index	10.611	5.019	6.935	4.554	9.608	6.595
Illegal Activities Index	0.104	0.048	0.093	0.055	0.097	0.060
Substance Frequency Index	0.143	0.137	0.108	0.124	0.171	0.152
Current Withdrawal Index	0.879	2.411	1.355	3.540	3.237	4.655
Treatment Resistance Index	0.968	0.960	0.935	0.894	1.495	1.159
Treatment Motivation Index	2.236	1.190	1.957	1.307	2.763	1.274
Self-Efficacy Index	4.465	0.955	4.500	1.009	3.546	1.377
Problem Orientation Index	0.764	1.581	1.051	1.695	1.381	1.864
Health Problem Index	0.134	0.152	0.210	0.158	0.126	0.149
Behavior Complexity Index	11.102	6.479	11.377	7.166	15.722	7.834
Emotional Problem Index	0.261	0.183	0.306	0.200	0.284	0.191
General Social Support Index	6.873	2.002	7.609	1.622	7.258	1.852
Training Activity Index	0.502	0.302	0.634	0.231	0.503	0.314
Recovery Environment Risk Index	0.288	0.080	0.279	0.093	0.355	0.109
Prior opiate use	0.229	0.420	0.123	0.329	0.515	0.500
Need for heroin treatment (self-reported)	0.025	0.158	0.000	0.000	0.000	0.000
Seizures/current withdrawal symptoms	0.025	0.158	0.080	0.271	0.196	0.397
Using daily	0.732	0.443	0.688	0.463	0.753	0.432
Using opioids[d]	0.083	0.276	0.058	0.234	0.206	0.405
Used in past two days	0.248	0.432	0.109	0.311	0.289	0.453
Substance use despite prior treatment	0.197	0.398	0.065	0.247	0.320	0.466
Acute health problems	0.338	0.473	0.609	0.488	0.361	0.480
High behavioral problems[a]	0.159	0.366	0.159	0.366	0.433	0.495
Days of victimization[c]	0.185	0.388	0.312	0.463	0.330	0.470
High victimization	0.471	0.499	0.435	0.496	0.691	0.462
Current criminal justice involvement	0.707	0.455	0.739	0.439	0.948	0.221
Total arrests[c]	0.389	0.674	0.478	0.651	0.588	1.063
Mental distress	0.280	0.449	0.362	0.481	0.361	0.480
High resistance	0.076	0.266	0.036	0.187	0.216	0.412
Low motivation	0.599	0.490	0.681	0.466	0.433	0.495
Low alc/drug use problem orientation	0.650	0.477	0.638	0.481	0.619	0.486
First high/intoxicated under age 15	0.879	0.326	0.775	0.417	0.979	0.142
Needle use[c]	0.013	0.112	0.007	0.085	0.010	0.101
In school	0.771	0.420	0.928	0.259	0.753	0.432
Employed	0.580	0.494	0.630	0.483	0.371	0.483
Homeless/runaway[a]	0.070	0.255	0.080	0.271	0.237	0.425
Family hist. of substance use	0.675	0.468	0.688	0.463	0.866	0.341
Weekly family problems[c]	0.229	0.420	0.384	0.486	0.340	0.474

Table A.3—Continued

Variables	Site H		Site I		Site J	
	Mean	SD	Mean	SD	Mean	SD
Drunk/high most of day[d]	13.395	20.632	9.572	16.822	22.247	25.273
Tobacco Dependence Index[b,e]	57.140	39.474	54.116	36.367	57.381	33.359
Health Distress Index[a]	1.599	0.970	1.601	1.004	1.660	1.083
Homicidal-Suicidal Thought Index	0.121	0.326	0.232	0.422	0.206	0.405
Lifetime detox admissions	0.115	0.852	0.014	0.120	0.072	0.259
Attended AA or other self-help	0.261	0.439	0.283	0.450	0.515	0.500
Last grade completed in school	9.408	1.387	9.275	1.172	8.763	1.242
Mention of alc as treatment need	0.089	0.285	0.159	0.366	0.124	0.329
Mention of marijuana as treatment need	0.592	0.491	0.529	0.499	0.474	0.499
Mention of cocaine as treatment need	0.038	0.192	0.007	0.085	0.082	0.275
Mention of opiates as treatment need	0.019	0.137	0.022	0.146	0.000	0.000
Mention of amph's as treatment need	0.000	0.000	0.007	0.085	0.155	0.362
Mention of other drugs as treatment need	0.019	0.137	0.065	0.247	0.041	0.199
Controlled environment[c]	10.051	22.150	10.935	21.721	22.485	24.365
Currently in alc/drug treatment	0.013	0.112	0.036	0.187	0.340	0.474
Gender						
Male	0.860	0.347	0.754	0.431	0.753	0.432
Female	0.140	0.347	0.246	0.431	0.247	0.432
Race						
Am. Indian	0.006	0.080	0.007	0.085	0.041	0.199
Black	0.217	0.412	0.101	0.302	0.062	0.241
White	0.713	0.452	0.797	0.402	0.485	0.500
Mexican	0.000	0.000	0.022	0.146	0.165	0.371
Other race	0.064	0.244	0.072	0.259	0.247	0.432
Substance most likes						
Alcohol	0.204	0.403	0.174	0.379	0.103	0.304
Cannabis	0.701	0.458	0.790	0.407	0.629	0.483
Crack or cocaine	0.032	0.176	0.000	0.000	0.041	0.199
Opiates	0.019	0.137	0.007	0.085	0.000	0.000
Hallucinogens	0.025	0.158	0.022	0.146	0.093	0.290
Amphetamines	0.000	0.000	0.007	0.085	0.134	0.341
Other substance	0.019	0.137	0.000	0.000	0.000	0.000
Current living status						
House/apt	0.834	0.372	0.957	0.204	0.794	0.405
Friend/relative	0.166	0.372	0.022	0.146	0.155	0.362
Jail/correctional	0.000	0.000	0.022	0.146	0.010	0.101
Other status	0.000	0.000	0.000	0.000	0.041	0.199

[a] Past year.

[b] Past month.

[c] Past 90 days.

[d] Weekly.

Table A.4
Baseline Covariate Differences Between Program and Comparison Groups Before and After Weighting: Site A

Variable	Unweighted				Weighted			
	Effect Size	P-value	KS Statistic	KS P-value	Effect Size	P-value	KS Statistic	KS P-value
Age	−0.061	0.687	0.123	0.110	−0.463	0.098	0.117	0.400
Times received treatment for drug/alc	−1.601	0.003	0.130	0.090	−1.845	0.025	0.134	0.240
Prior treatment psychological problems	1.008	0.000	0.469	0.000	0.502	0.010	0.233	0.020
No. people lived with[a]	0.179	0.192	0.199	0.000	−0.020	0.914	0.137	0.230
Substance Dependence Index[a]	0.593	0.000	0.233	0.010	0.040	0.834	0.079	0.760
Substance Dependence Index[b]	−0.382	0.013	0.139	0.080	−0.611	0.013	0.204	0.000
Drug Crime Index, minus L3t	0.492	0.001	0.256	0.000	0.197	0.281	0.136	0.220
Living Risk Index	0.629	0.000	0.290	0.000	0.201	0.289	0.120	0.410
Vocational Risk Index	0.392	0.007	0.241	0.000	0.086	0.670	0.075	0.930
Social Risk Index	0.528	0.000	0.261	0.000	0.221	0.322	0.132	0.290
Needle Frequency Index	−0.909	0.000	0.245	0.000	−0.502	0.021	0.159	0.040
Needle Problem Index	−0.021	0.885	0.019	0.810	0.076	0.595	0.024	0.530
Sex Protection Ratio	0.005	0.974	0.053	0.890	0.103	0.602	0.091	0.690
Controlled Environment Index	1.470	0.000	0.587	0.000	0.688	0.001	0.329	0.010
General Satisfaction Index	0.034	0.819	0.059	0.980	0.056	0.799	0.089	0.720
Mental Health Treatment Index	0.323	0.017	0.267	0.000	0.117	0.554	0.171	0.040
Criminal Justice System Index	0.970	0.000	0.361	0.000	0.717	0.001	0.268	0.020
Training Problem Index	0.040	0.789	0.113	0.310	0.150	0.505	0.126	0.340
Substance Abuse Treatment Index	−0.025	0.867	0.046	0.790	−0.532	0.129	0.112	0.430
Substance Problem Index[a]	0.785	0.000	0.290	0.000	0.239	0.231	0.105	0.560
Substance Problem Index[b]	−0.288	0.053	0.155	0.080	−0.454	0.041	0.191	0.100
Physical Health Treatment Index	0.112	0.449	0.150	0.070	−0.088	0.688	0.091	0.580
Internal Mental Distress Index	0.388	0.006	0.172	0.060	0.097	0.586	0.069	0.950
Environmental Risk Index	0.726	0.000	0.324	0.000	0.264	0.208	0.131	0.440
General Victimization Index	0.102	0.455	0.213	0.000	0.018	0.923	0.088	0.720
Personal Sources of Stress Index	0.514	0.000	0.273	0.000	0.187	0.313	0.103	0.470
Other Sources of Stress Index	0.498	0.000	0.212	0.000	0.311	0.103	0.150	0.150
Employment Problem Index	0.293	0.035	0.214	0.000	0.121	0.484	0.088	0.440
Employment Activity Index	−0.057	0.695	0.081	0.450	−0.045	0.818	0.103	0.280
Crime Violence Index	0.418	0.004	0.249	0.000	0.212	0.257	0.142	0.320
Illegal Activities Index	0.362	0.017	0.214	0.010	0.157	0.465	0.171	0.160
Substance Frequency Index	−0.445	0.004	0.245	0.000	−0.139	0.524	0.196	0.140

Table A.4—Continued

Variable	Unweighted				Weighted			
	Effect Size	P-value	KS Statistic	KS P-value	Effect Size	P-value	KS Statistic	KS P-value
Current Withdrawal Index	−0.387	0.012	0.144	0.010	−0.288	0.120	0.149	0.090
Treatment Resistance Index	0.202	0.161	0.092	0.280	0.038	0.836	0.026	0.970
Treatment Motivation Index	0.970	0.000	0.322	0.000	0.318	0.081	0.110	0.290
Self-Efficacy Index	−0.200	0.156	0.138	0.110	−0.220	0.185	0.143	0.190
Problem Orientation Index	0.674	0.000	0.343	0.000	0.272	0.160	0.167	0.120
Health Problem Index	0.406	0.005	0.298	0.000	0.300	0.086	0.222	0.070
Behavior Complexity Index	0.575	0.000	0.206	0.010	0.240	0.240	0.136	0.440
Emotional Problem Index	0.375	0.007	0.208	0.030	0.134	0.431	0.099	0.820
General Social Support Index	0.476	0.001	0.167	0.060	0.231	0.238	0.094	0.660
Training Activity Index	0.614	0.000	0.204	0.000	0.429	0.061	0.171	0.240
Recovery Environment Risk Index	0.122	0.393	0.150	0.160	−0.088	0.654	0.077	0.960
Prior opiate use	0.321	0.023	0.153	0.020	0.168	0.358	0.080	0.290
Need for heroin treatment (self-reported)	NA	0.000	0.045	0.100	NA	0.072	0.019	0.130
Seizures/current withdrawal symptoms	−0.216	0.161	0.040	0.200	−0.058	0.754	0.011	0.760
Using daily	−0.410	0.004	0.202	0.000	−0.239	0.187	0.118	0.210
Using opioids[d]	0.190	0.179	0.084	0.150	0.098	0.593	0.043	0.610
Used in past two days	−0.049	0.740	0.006	0.750	−0.240	0.330	0.032	0.390
Substance use despite prior treatment	−0.007	0.959	0.002	0.960	−0.147	0.457	0.041	0.460
Acute health problems	0.194	0.174	0.095	0.110	0.187	0.295	0.092	0.370
High behavioral problems[a]	0.331	0.020	0.165	0.010	0.076	0.681	0.038	0.590
Days of victimization[c]	−0.129	0.376	0.049	0.430	−0.273	0.172	0.104	0.190
High victimization	−0.054	0.709	0.026	0.720	−0.034	0.853	0.017	0.770
Current criminal justice involvement	−0.122	0.379	0.031	0.230	0.195	0.416	0.050	0.300
Total arrests[c]	0.401	0.004	0.236	0.000	0.214	0.277	0.210	0.020
Mental distress	0.432	0.002	0.216	0.000	0.210	0.257	0.105	0.220
High resistance	0.080	0.573	0.029	0.520	−0.025	0.899	0.009	0.880
Low motivation	−0.739	0.000	0.301	0.000	−0.097	0.580	0.039	0.630
Low alc/drug use problem orientation	−0.637	0.000	0.292	0.000	−0.307	0.109	0.140	0.170
First high/intoxicated under age 15	0.444	0.007	0.082	0.080	0.650	0.032	0.120	0.030
Needle use[c]	−0.956	0.000	0.244	0.000	−0.591	0.011	0.151	0.030
In school	1.013	0.000	0.186	0.000	0.793	0.010	0.146	0.010
Employed	0.014	0.921	0.006	0.920	0.036	0.844	0.015	0.890
Homeless/runaway[a]	0.321	0.023	0.153	0.000	0.059	0.754	0.028	0.780
Family hist. of substance use	0.632	0.000	0.179	0.000	0.365	0.080	0.103	0.120
Weekly family problems[c]	−0.068	0.636	0.033	0.620	0.098	0.584	0.048	0.530
Drunk/high most of day[d]	−0.279	0.072	0.181	0.070	−0.165	0.453	0.174	0.230

Table A.4—Continued

Variable	Unweighted				Weighted			
	Effect Size	P-value	KS Statistic	KS P-value	Effect Size	P-value	KS Statistic	KS P-value
Tobacco Dependence Index[b,e]	−0.457	0.003	0.328	0.000	−0.293	0.166	0.254	0.060
Health Distress Index[a]	0.322	0.026	0.134	0.080	0.212	0.262	0.099	0.340
Homicidal-Suicidal Thought Index	0.020	0.887	0.008	0.910	0.110	0.508	0.042	0.480
Lifetime detox admissions	−2.854	0.000	0.147	0.000	−2.089	0.001	0.156	0.000
Attended AA or other self-help	0.791	0.000	0.332	0.000	0.422	0.033	0.177	0.080
Last grade completed in school	0.056	0.702	0.041	0.880	−0.250	0.220	0.139	0.240
Mention of alc as treatment need	0.633	0.000	0.311	0.000	0.272	0.142	0.133	0.110
Mention of marijuana as treatment need	0.581	0.000	0.285	0.000	0.183	0.325	0.090	0.320
Mention of cocaine as treatment need	−0.368	0.020	0.082	0.100	−0.266	0.246	0.059	0.180
Mention of opiates as treatment need	NA	0.000	0.045	0.100	NA	0.072	0.019	0.130
Mention of amph's as treatment need	0.369	0.008	0.159	0.000	0.223	0.204	0.096	0.120
Mention of other drugs as treatment need	0.274	0.045	0.090	0.010	0.288	0.041	0.095	0.050
Controlled environment[c]	0.950	0.000	0.523	0.000	0.222	0.297	0.242	0.050
Currently in alc/drug treatment	0.192	0.175	0.086	0.180	0.200	0.258	0.090	0.170
Gender								
Male	−0.422	0.743	0.201	0.000	−0.143	0.917	0.068	0.440
Female	0.422	NA	0.201	0.000	0.143	NA	0.068	0.440
Race								
Am. Indian	NA	NA	0.018	0.270	NA	NA	0.033	0.270
Black	0.230	NA	0.096	0.070	0.180	NA	0.075	0.350
White	0.474	NA	0.235	0.000	0.346	NA	0.172	0.050
Mexican	−0.896	0.991	0.275	0.000	−0.472	0.997	0.145	0.080
Other race	−0.092	NA	0.038	0.590	−0.165	NA	0.069	0.390
Substance most likes								
Alcohol	0.223	NA	0.091	0.010	0.028	NA	0.012	0.870
Cannabis	−0.200	NA	0.100	0.170	0.055	NA	0.027	0.780
Crack or cocaine	−0.297	1.000	0.055	0.130	−0.321	1.000	0.059	0.180
Opiates	NA	NA	0.042	0.120	NA	NA	0.014	0.440
Hallucinogens	0.077	NA	0.014	0.580	0.010	NA	0.002	0.870
Amphetamines	0.244	NA	0.089	0.010	0.052	NA	0.019	0.810
Other substance	0.020	NA	0.003	0.880	0.102	NA	0.013	0.670
Current living status								
House/apt	−0.327	0.996	0.163	0.010	0.019	NA	0.009	0.910
Friend/relative	0.131	NA	0.050	0.290	0.037	NA	0.014	0.740
Jail/correctional	0.060	NA	0.018	0.700	−0.112	1.000	0.035	0.570
Other status	0.249	NA	0.095	0.020	0.029	NA	0.011	0.870

Table A.4—Continued

	N	Effective Sample Size	Average Effect Size	Max Effect Size	Average KS Statistic	Max KS Statistic	KS P-value
Unweighted	XXX[e]	XXX[e]	0.416	2.854	0.165	0.587	0.000
Weighted	XXX[e]	61.502	0.256	2.089	0.102	0.329	0.040

[a] Past year.

[b] Past month.

[c] Past 90 days.

[d] Weekly.

[e] Sample sizes censored in these tables to preserve program anonymity. For available sample sizes, see Table A.1.

Table A.5
Baseline Covariate Differences Between Program and Comparison Groups Before and After Weighting: Site B

Variable	Unweighted				Weighted			
	Effect Size	P-value	KS Statistic	KS P-value	Effect Size	P-value	KS Statistic	KS P-value
Age	−0.390	0.008	0.133	0.000	−0.106	0.486	0.063	0.470
Times received treatment for drug/alc	0.167	0.045	0.086	0.170	0.110	0.243	0.056	0.690
Prior treatment psychological problems	−0.388	0.001	0.152	0.000	−0.119	0.325	0.047	0.380
No. people lived with[a]	−0.070	0.518	0.097	0.100	0.051	0.569	0.028	1.000
Substance Dependence Index[a]	0.094	0.391	0.116	0.030	0.101	0.445	0.076	0.530
Substance Dependence Index[b]	0.269	0.008	0.168	0.000	0.187	0.139	0.093	0.370
Drug Crime Index, minus L3t	−0.176	0.110	0.080	0.140	0.032	0.802	0.054	0.520
Living Risk Index	−0.447	0.000	0.151	0.010	−0.077	0.534	0.042	0.970
Vocational Risk Index	−0.066	0.529	0.076	0.450	−0.004	0.975	0.046	0.960
Social Risk Index	−0.138	0.202	0.136	0.040	−0.144	0.278	0.115	0.200
Needle Frequency Index	0.317	0.005	0.223	0.000	0.251	0.052	0.167	0.010
Needle Problem Index	−0.185	0.152	0.029	0.330	−0.081	0.494	0.016	0.790
Sex Protection Ratio	−0.001	0.989	0.028	0.970	−0.032	0.815	0.045	0.870
Controlled Environment Index	−0.651	0.000	0.237	0.000	−0.250	0.053	0.105	0.300
General Satisfaction Index	0.106	0.320	0.059	0.680	0.060	0.628	0.060	0.830
Mental Health Treatment Index	−0.286	0.052	0.075	0.040	−0.146	0.288	0.029	0.570
Criminal Justice System Index	−0.103	0.317	0.078	0.340	−0.042	0.746	0.041	0.750
Training Problem Index	0.254	0.027	0.097	0.120	0.140	0.318	0.057	0.770
Substance Abuse Treatment Index	−0.071	0.538	0.033	0.730	−0.001	0.993	0.058	0.480
Substance Problem Index[a]	0.149	0.198	0.138	0.010	0.149	0.266	0.084	0.520
Substance Problem Index[b]	0.323	0.002	0.218	0.000	0.232	0.054	0.130	0.190
Physical Health Treatment Index	−0.070	0.516	0.051	0.610	0.040	0.705	0.056	0.610

Table A.5—Continued

Variable	Unweighted				Weighted			
	Effect Size	P-value	KS Statistic	KS P-value	Effect Size	P-value	KS Statistic	KS P-value
Internal Mental Distress Index	−0.226	0.039	0.117	0.040	0.015	0.900	0.068	0.780
Environmental Risk Index	−0.231	0.039	0.134	0.010	−0.096	0.474	0.083	0.510
General Victimization Index	−0.243	0.048	0.162	0.000	−0.021	0.867	0.059	0.630
Personal Sources of Stress Index	−0.398	0.000	0.178	0.000	−0.133	0.285	0.081	0.370
Other Sources of Stress Index	−0.186	0.077	0.109	0.040	0.010	0.932	0.035	0.970
Employment Problem Index	−0.419	0.002	0.099	0.050	−0.144	0.231	0.050	0.410
Employment Activity Index	−0.014	0.892	0.050	0.480	0.005	0.966	0.039	0.910
Crime Violence Index	−0.351	0.002	0.158	0.000	−0.123	0.348	0.085	0.510
Illegal Activities Index	−0.161	0.109	0.089	0.280	−0.055	0.672	0.061	0.830
Substance Frequency Index	0.194	0.078	0.150	0.010	0.105	0.430	0.113	0.450
Current Withdrawal Index	−0.117	0.290	0.049	0.640	−0.028	0.803	0.051	0.710
Treatment Resistance Index	−0.269	0.014	0.089	0.080	−0.045	0.710	0.038	0.830
Treatment Motivation Index	0.287	0.010	0.176	0.000	0.260	0.052	0.153	0.050
Self-Efficacy Index	0.104	0.343	0.049	0.630	0.001	0.993	0.043	0.840
Problem Orientation Index	0.056	0.589	0.046	0.440	0.187	0.106	0.107	0.090
Health Problem Index	0.014	0.901	0.093	0.260	0.087	0.497	0.130	0.150
Behavior Complexity Index	−0.294	0.008	0.219	0.000	−0.073	0.570	0.084	0.570
Emotional Problem Index	−0.168	0.141	0.079	0.460	0.016	0.901	0.080	0.710
General Social Support Index	0.015	0.887	0.037	0.860	0.092	0.490	0.064	0.710
Training Activity Index	0.113	0.291	0.079	0.580	0.064	0.606	0.085	0.670
Recovery Environment Risk Index	0.109	0.308	0.090	0.340	0.180	0.103	0.120	0.250
Prior opiate use	−0.151	0.164	0.058	0.170	−0.022	0.860	0.008	0.880
Need for heroin treatment (self-reported)	−0.219	0.093	0.030	0.090	−0.066	0.566	0.009	0.710
Seizures/current withdrawal symptoms	0.021	0.838	0.005	0.760	0.139	0.139	0.036	0.240
Using daily	0.369	0.001	0.137	0.000	0.252	0.064	0.093	0.070
Using opioids[d]	−0.090	0.399	0.034	0.460	−0.013	0.917	0.005	0.930
Used in past two days	−0.142	0.260	0.016	0.280	−0.150	0.312	0.017	0.310
Substance use despite prior treatment	0.050	0.619	0.015	0.550	0.035	0.773	0.010	0.880
Acute health problems	0.200	0.049	0.097	0.070	0.213	0.074	0.103	0.060
High behavioral problems[a]	−0.555	0.000	0.221	0.000	−0.239	0.074	0.095	0.080
Days of victimization[c]	0.238	0.016	0.107	0.020	0.129	0.319	0.058	0.260
High victimization	−0.218	0.033	0.108	0.030	−0.132	0.290	0.066	0.290
Current criminal justice involvement	∞	0.000	0.071	0.000	∞	0.003	0.051	0.000
Total arrests[c]	−0.088	0.408	0.043	0.580	−0.003	0.982	0.018	0.980
Mental distress	−0.242	0.026	0.104	0.020	−0.020	0.869	0.008	0.790
High resistance	−0.188	0.097	0.056	0.140	−0.021	0.864	0.006	0.820
Low motivation	−0.291	0.006	0.141	0.000	−0.319	0.015	0.155	0.040

Table A.5—Continued

Variable	Unweighted				Weighted			
	Effect Size	P-value	KS Statistic	KS P-value	Effect Size	P-value	KS Statistic	KS P-value
Low alc/drug use problem orientation	0.061	0.558	0.030	0.440	−0.139	0.252	0.069	0.220
First high/intoxicated under age 15	0.034	0.749	0.010	0.820	−0.046	0.679	0.014	0.720
Needle use[c]	0.409	0.000	0.200	0.000	0.324	0.008	0.159	0.000
In school	0.101	0.345	0.038	0.410	0.022	0.860	0.008	0.820
Employed	0.011	0.912	0.005	0.940	0.019	0.885	0.008	0.890
Homeless/runaway[a]	−0.011	0.914	0.005	0.940	0.073	0.528	0.030	0.540
Family hist. of substance use	0.092	0.385	0.038	0.410	0.121	0.365	0.050	0.370
Weekly family problems[c]	0.194	0.059	0.097	0.060	0.138	0.280	0.069	0.340
Drunk/high most of day[d]	0.128	0.213	0.105	0.160	0.070	0.576	0.071	0.830
Tobacco Dependence Index[b,e]	0.106	0.305	0.079	0.350	0.155	0.207	0.093	0.400
Health Distress Index[a]	0.031	0.763	0.021	0.970	−0.012	0.928	0.014	0.990
Homicidal-Suicidal Thought Index	−0.080	0.456	0.029	0.470	−0.047	0.702	0.017	0.750
Lifetime detox admissions	−0.138	0.418	0.013	0.920	0.070	0.508	0.028	0.690
Attended AA or other self-help	0.016	0.877	0.008	0.850	0.088	0.492	0.044	0.440
Last grade completed in school	0.106	0.339	0.067	0.310	0.058	0.662	0.079	0.340
Mention of alc as treatment need	−0.547	0.000	0.129	0.000	−0.186	0.150	0.044	0.250
Mention of marijuana as treatment need	−0.037	0.720	0.018	0.770	0.039	0.764	0.018	0.730
Mention of cocaine as treatment need	0.158	0.106	0.057	0.090	0.161	0.135	0.059	0.230
Mention of opiates as treatment need	−0.219	0.093	0.030	0.090	−0.066	0.566	0.009	0.710
Mention of amph's as treatment need	0.290	0.002	0.111	0.000	0.317	0.001	0.121	0.010
Mention of other drugs as treatment need	−0.472	0.004	0.054	0.000	−0.249	0.077	0.028	0.200
Controlled environment[c]	−0.461	0.000	0.223	0.000	−0.140	0.255	0.094	0.360
Currently in alc/drug treatment	−0.068	0.520	0.027	0.560	−0.048	0.720	0.019	0.700
Gender								
Male	0.035	NA	0.013	0.740	−0.082	NA	0.031	0.550
Female	−0.035	0.981	0.013	0.740	0.082	0.952	0.031	0.550
Race								
Am. Indian	0.161	NA	0.029	0.030	0.117	NA	0.021	0.270
Black	−0.405	0.998	0.109	0.010	−0.265	1.000	0.072	0.070
White	−0.138	NA	0.055	0.190	0.017	NA	0.007	0.900
Mexican	0.374	NA	0.186	0.000	0.066	NA	0.033	0.650
Other race	−0.119	NA	0.050	0.310	0.027	NA	0.011	0.880
Substance most likes								
Alcohol	−0.231	NA	0.067	0.060	−0.115	NA	0.033	0.440

Table A.5—Continued

Variable	Unweighted Effect Size	P-value	KS Statistic	KS P-value	Weighted Effect Size	P-value	KS Statistic	KS P-value
Cannabis	−0.080	NA	0.039	0.460	−0.194	NA	0.095	0.130
Crack or cocaine	0.213	NA	0.071	0.010	0.210	NA	0.070	0.070
Opiates	−0.325	1.000	0.037	0.010	−0.122	NA	0.014	0.370
Hallucinogens	−0.039	NA	0.005	0.810	−0.041	NA	0.006	0.790
Amphetamines	0.241	NA	0.081	0.000	0.251	1.000	0.085	0.020
Other substance	−0.031	NA	0.004	0.720	−0.058	NA	0.007	0.760
Current living status								
House/apt	0.254	NA	0.110	0.030	0.066	NA	0.029	0.580
Friend/relative	−0.040	NA	0.013	0.730	0.023	NA	0.008	0.840
Jail/correctional	−0.064	NA	0.017	0.640	0.004	NA	0.001	0.950
Other status	−0.379	0.997	0.079	0.000	−0.177	1.000	0.037	0.240

	N	Effective Sample Size	Average Effect Size	Max Effect Size	Average KS Statistic	Max KS Statistic	KS P-value
Unweighted	XXX[e]	XXX[e]	0.189	0.651	0.083	0.237	0.000
Weighted	XXX[e]	102.583	0.105	0.324	0.056	0.167	0.620

[a] Past year.

[b] Past month.

[c] Past 90 days.

[d] Weekly.

[e] Sample sizes censored in these tables to preserve program anonymity. For available sample sizes, see Table A.1.

Table A.6
Baseline Covariate Differences Between Program and Comparison Groups Before and After Weighting: Site C

Variable	Unweighted Effect Size	P-value	KS Statistic	KS P-value	Weighted Effect Size	P-value	KS Statistic	KS P-value
Age	0.890	0.000	0.489	0.000	0.802	0.000	0.481	0.000
Times received treatment for drug/alc	−0.194	0.344	0.209	0.000	−0.864	0.233	0.123	0.460
Prior treatment psychological problems	0.165	0.257	0.079	0.300	−0.043	0.833	0.021	0.850
No. people lived with[a]	−0.157	0.351	0.098	0.310	−0.303	0.397	0.103	0.630
Substance Dependence Index[a]	0.985	0.000	0.407	0.000	0.412	0.038	0.279	0.000
Substance Dependence Index[b]	0.666	0.000	0.329	0.000	0.288	0.121	0.164	0.250
Drug Crime Index, minus L3t	0.487	0.001	0.213	0.010	0.119	0.551	0.074	0.770
Living Risk Index	0.114	0.432	0.114	0.340	−0.079	0.766	0.069	0.970
Vocational Risk Index	−0.087	0.549	0.139	0.190	−0.237	0.266	0.160	0.370
Social Risk Index	0.110	0.442	0.164	0.060	−0.048	0.799	0.101	0.820
Needle Frequency Index	0.193	0.164	0.142	0.040	0.250	0.092	0.142	0.220
Needle Problem Index	0.423	0.002	0.186	0.000	0.362	0.021	0.153	0.050

Table A.6—Continued

Variable	Unweighted				Weighted			
	Effect Size	P-value	KS Statistic	KS P-value	Effect Size	P-value	KS Statistic	KS P-value
Sex Protection Ratio	−0.223	0.123	0.146	0.090	−0.221	0.215	0.129	0.460
Controlled Environment Index	−0.042	0.777	0.152	0.120	0.162	0.414	0.306	0.000
General Satisfaction Index	−0.353	0.014	0.174	0.100	−0.321	0.115	0.133	0.580
Mental Health Treatment Index	−0.483	0.012	0.100	0.030	−0.454	0.100	0.117	0.050
Criminal Justice System Index	−0.726	0.000	0.356	0.000	−0.397	0.078	0.238	0.050
Training Problem Index	−0.610	0.000	0.398	0.000	−0.547	0.002	0.315	0.000
Substance Abuse Treatment Index	0.237	0.095	0.208	0.000	0.008	0.969	0.118	0.420
Substance Problem Index[a]	0.836	0.000	0.383	0.000	0.287	0.121	0.240	0.020
Substance Problem Index[b]	0.648	0.000	0.323	0.000	0.293	0.126	0.170	0.280
Physical Health Treatment Index	0.164	0.238	0.112	0.220	0.083	0.595	0.171	0.150
Internal Mental Distress Index	0.656	0.000	0.260	0.000	0.244	0.225	0.149	0.520
Environmental Risk Index	0.026	0.858	0.091	0.620	−0.194	0.407	0.112	0.790
General Victimization Index	0.437	0.002	0.366	0.000	0.276	0.158	0.184	0.200
Personal Sources of Stress Index	0.424	0.004	0.210	0.010	0.130	0.564	0.122	0.480
Other Sources of Stress Index	0.261	0.077	0.166	0.020	0.085	0.698	0.152	0.270
Employment Problem Index	0.595	0.000	0.326	0.000	0.625	0.000	0.344	0.000
Employment Activity Index	0.143	0.322	0.136	0.060	0.103	0.576	0.156	0.180
Crime Violence Index	0.463	0.001	0.265	0.000	0.207	0.346	0.179	0.340
Illegal Activities Index	0.121	0.400	0.150	0.140	−0.085	0.673	0.148	0.500
Substance Frequency Index	0.754	0.000	0.365	0.000	0.080	0.690	0.135	0.630
Current Withdrawal Index	0.663	0.000	0.351	0.000	0.310	0.106	0.167	0.290
Treatment Resistance Index	0.532	0.000	0.199	0.000	0.343	0.074	0.119	0.500
Treatment Motivation Index	1.022	0.000	0.285	0.000	0.232	0.366	0.119	0.400
Self-Efficacy Index	−0.525	0.000	0.233	0.000	−0.209	0.315	0.124	0.450
Problem Orientation Index	0.577	0.000	0.274	0.000	0.289	0.140	0.186	0.120
Health Problem Index	0.119	0.398	0.088	0.640	0.122	0.472	0.081	0.860
Behavior Complexity Index	0.570	0.000	0.268	0.000	0.235	0.292	0.159	0.410
Emotional Problem Index	0.384	0.008	0.216	0.030	−0.033	0.883	0.088	0.950
General Social Support Index	−0.167	0.252	0.112	0.250	−0.134	0.507	0.103	0.680
Training Activity Index	−1.121	0.000	0.493	0.000	−0.623	0.005	0.307	0.020
Recovery Environment Risk Index	0.419	0.005	0.244	0.010	−0.232	0.423	0.172	0.340
Prior opiate use	0.738	0.000	0.368	0.000	0.493	0.011	0.246	0.010
Need for heroin treatment (self-reported)	0.513	0.000	0.213	0.000	0.521	0.000	0.216	0.010
Seizures/current withdrawal symptoms	0.466	0.001	0.199	0.000	0.308	0.065	0.132	0.080
Using daily	0.326	0.033	0.116	0.080	−0.141	0.406	0.050	0.420

Table A.6—Continued

Variable	Unweighted				Weighted			
	Effect Size	P-value	KS Statistic	KS P-value	Effect Size	P-value	KS Statistic	KS P-value
Using opioids[d]	0.759	0.000	0.379	0.000	0.468	0.015	0.234	0.010
Used in past two days	0.278	0.044	0.081	0.010	0.232	0.126	0.067	0.150
Substance use despite prior treatment	0.329	0.020	0.132	0.010	0.010	0.960	0.004	0.930
Acute health problems	−0.115	0.436	0.052	0.490	−0.051	0.798	0.023	0.780
High behavioral problems[a]	0.567	0.000	0.280	0.000	0.205	0.328	0.102	0.310
Days of victimization[c]	0.111	0.446	0.049	0.430	0.111	0.568	0.048	0.580
High victimization	0.381	0.011	0.163	0.010	0.242	0.266	0.103	0.260
Current criminal justice involvement	−0.535	0.000	0.229	0.000	−0.384	0.031	0.164	0.040
Total arrests[c]	−0.483	0.002	0.218	0.010	−0.436	0.056	0.185	0.050
Mental distress	0.581	0.000	0.288	0.000	0.308	0.136	0.153	0.140
High resistance	0.415	0.003	0.189	0.000	0.260	0.204	0.119	0.160
Low motivation	−0.761	0.000	0.307	0.000	−0.191	0.406	0.077	0.330
Low alc/drug use problem orientation	−0.330	0.025	0.162	0.020	−0.128	0.541	0.063	0.530
First high/intoxicated under age 15	−0.192	0.179	0.072	0.090	−0.216	0.223	0.081	0.310
Needle use[c]	−0.216	0.149	0.087	0.160	0.012	0.951	0.005	0.950
In school	−0.797	0.000	0.398	0.000	−0.495	0.017	0.247	0.010
Employed	0.097	0.507	0.043	0.490	0.054	0.781	0.024	0.770
Homeless/runaway[a]	−0.104	0.484	0.040	0.480	−0.054	0.787	0.021	0.770
Family hist. of substance use	−0.001	0.995	0.000	0.990	−0.030	0.886	0.013	0.900
Weekly family problems[c]	0.375	0.011	0.185	0.000	−0.079	0.688	0.039	0.700
Drunk/high most of day[d]	0.503	0.001	0.278	0.000	−0.011	0.958	0.171	0.300
Tobacco Dependence Index[b,e]	2.245	0.000	0.668	0.000	0.589	0.017	0.213	0.000
Health Distress Index[a]	0.332	0.023	0.158	0.080	0.081	0.680	0.063	0.850
Homicidal-Suicidal Thought Index	0.324	0.024	0.148	0.010	0.427	0.006	0.195	0.010
Lifetime detox admissions	0.297	0.031	0.221	0.000	0.256	0.078	0.187	0.020
Attended AA or other self-help	−0.147	0.319	0.073	0.360	−0.185	0.375	0.092	0.440
Last grade completed in school	0.413	0.004	0.170	0.030	0.512	0.009	0.172	0.150
Mention of alc as treatment need	0.279	0.051	0.119	0.020	0.098	0.632	0.042	0.560
Mention of marijuana as treatment need	0.384	0.009	0.192	0.010	0.187	0.358	0.094	0.390
Mention of cocaine as treatment need	0.441	0.002	0.201	0.000	0.329	0.071	0.150	0.050
Mention of opiates as treatment need	0.513	0.000	0.213	0.000	0.521	0.000	0.216	0.010
Mention of amph's as treatment need	−0.787	0.000	0.106	0.010	−1.410	0.003	0.190	0.010
Mention of other drugs as treatment need	0.333	0.017	0.118	0.000	0.153	0.445	0.054	0.440

Table A.6—Continued

Variable	Unweighted				Weighted			
	Effect Size	P-value	KS Statistic	KS P-value	Effect Size	P-value	KS Statistic	KS P-value
Controlled environment[c]	−0.077	0.601	0.150	0.130	0.134	0.496	0.293	0.000
Currently in alc/drug treatment	0.042	0.774	0.017	0.770	0.103	0.606	0.043	0.610
Gender								
Male	−0.256	0.845	0.115	0.050	−0.029	0.983	0.013	0.900
Female	0.256	NA	0.115	0.050	0.029	NA	0.013	0.900
Race								
Am. Indian	0.027	NA	0.004	0.800	−0.075	NA	0.010	0.750
Black	0.008	NA	0.003	0.980	−0.156	NA	0.056	0.560
White	0.277	NA	0.132	0.010	0.151	NA	0.072	0.440
Mexican	NA	NA	0.395	0.000	NA	NA	0.134	0.000
Other race	0.512	0.972	0.256	0.000	0.257	0.996	0.128	0.220
Substance most likes								
Alcohol	−0.162	NA	0.047	0.270	0.103	NA	0.030	0.590
Cannabis	−0.343	NA	0.171	0.020	−0.303	NA	0.151	0.190
Crack or cocaine	0.165	NA	0.055	0.170	0.028	NA	0.009	0.920
Opiates	0.520	NA	0.216	0.000	0.529	NA	0.220	0.010
Hallucinogens	0.165	NA	0.038	0.090	−0.013	NA	0.003	0.990
Amphetamines	−0.545	0.999	0.073	0.100	−0.735	0.999	0.099	0.050
Other substance	NA	NA	0.018	0.250	NA	NA	0.006	0.180
Current living status								
House/apt	0.265	NA	0.110	0.170	0.378	NA	0.157	0.060
Friend/relative	−0.392	0.997	0.090	0.040	−0.401	0.992	0.092	0.080
Jail/correctional	0.012	NA	0.004	0.920	0.091	NA	0.027	0.590
Other status	−0.091	NA	0.024	0.630	−0.351	NA	0.092	0.120

	N	Effective Sample Size	Average Effect Size	Max Effect Size	Average KS Statistic	Max KS Statistic	KS P-value
Unweighted	XXX[e]	XXX[e]	0.402	2.245	0.190	0.668	0.000
Weighted	XXX[e]	41.627	0.259	1.410	0.130	0.481	0.000

[a] Past year.

[b] Past month.

[c] Past 90 days.

[d] Weekly.

[e] Sample sizes censored in these tables to preserve program anonymity. For available sample sizes, see Table A.1.

Table A.7
Baseline Covariate Differences Between Program and Comparison Groups Before and After Weighting: Site D

Variable	Unweighted				Weighted			
	Effect Size	P-value	KS Statistic	KS P-value	Effect Size	P-value	KS Statistic	KS P-value
Age	0.473	0.000	0.201	0.000	0.277	0.030	0.159	0.010
Times received treatment for drug/alc	0.401	0.000	0.264	0.000	0.040	0.909	0.197	0.010
Prior treatment psychological problems	0.292	0.002	0.145	0.000	0.030	0.824	0.015	0.820
No. people lived with[a]	−0.025	0.794	0.102	0.040	0.053	0.675	0.078	0.570
Substance Dependence Index[a]	0.312	0.001	0.144	0.010	0.245	0.109	0.107	0.170
Substance Dependence Index[b]	0.278	0.002	0.166	0.000	0.174	0.175	0.124	0.170
Drug Crime Index, minus L3t	0.329	0.001	0.147	0.000	0.128	0.309	0.093	0.290
Living Risk Index	−0.131	0.156	0.124	0.020	0.034	0.789	0.073	0.710
Vocational Risk Index	−0.494	0.000	0.255	0.000	−0.411	0.002	0.208	0.000
Social Risk Index	0.127	0.173	0.091	0.160	0.040	0.767	0.054	0.980
Needle Frequency Index	0.457	0.000	0.206	0.000	0.460	0.000	0.203	0.000
Needle Problem Index	0.471	0.000	0.210	0.000	0.461	0.000	0.205	0.000
Sex Protection Ratio	−0.370	0.000	0.265	0.000	−0.298	0.023	0.233	0.010
Controlled Environment Index	0.200	0.034	0.182	0.000	0.181	0.197	0.161	0.090
General Satisfaction Index	−0.131	0.153	0.111	0.070	−0.027	0.818	0.090	0.490
Mental Health Treatment Index	0.067	0.446	0.029	0.760	−0.064	0.619	0.101	0.120
Criminal Justice System Index	0.207	0.031	0.140	0.010	0.077	0.577	0.091	0.330
Training Problem Index	−0.349	0.000	0.201	0.000	−0.169	0.204	0.111	0.340
Substance Abuse Treatment Index	−0.022	0.830	0.070	0.300	0.020	0.882	0.047	0.900
Substance Problem Index[a]	0.261	0.006	0.142	0.010	0.183	0.174	0.140	0.080
Substance Problem Index[b]	0.234	0.010	0.204	0.000	0.093	0.448	0.124	0.220
Physical Health Treatment Index	0.069	0.428	0.082	0.100	0.009	0.925	0.132	0.060
Internal Mental Distress Index	−0.117	0.211	0.093	0.190	−0.149	0.271	0.098	0.430
Environmental Risk Index	−0.313	0.001	0.158	0.000	−0.241	0.059	0.169	0.070
General Victimization Index	−0.082	0.388	0.087	0.210	−0.107	0.433	0.086	0.560
Personal Sources of Stress Index	−0.061	0.519	0.035	0.760	−0.140	0.263	0.083	0.460
Other Sources of Stress Index	−0.073	0.433	0.111	0.020	−0.227	0.092	0.133	0.090
Employment Problem Index	0.538	0.000	0.268	0.000	0.262	0.038	0.146	0.120
Employment Activity Index	0.341	0.000	0.166	0.000	0.052	0.686	0.103	0.440
Crime Violence Index	0.464	0.000	0.218	0.000	0.267	0.040	0.164	0.070
Illegal Activities Index	0.316	0.001	0.125	0.010	0.056	0.643	0.076	0.780
Substance Frequency Index	0.672	0.000	0.249	0.000	0.293	0.018	0.128	0.220
Current Withdrawal Index	0.039	0.666	0.064	0.370	0.165	0.132	0.101	0.240

Table A.7—Continued

Variable	Unweighted				Weighted			
	Effect Size	P-value	KS Statistic	KS P-value	Effect Size	P-value	KS Statistic	KS P-value
Treatment Resistance Index	−0.348	0.000	0.132	0.000	−0.220	0.124	0.086	0.340
Treatment Motivation Index	0.057	0.546	0.039	0.670	0.018	0.890	0.033	0.880
Self-Efficacy Index	0.161	0.098	0.058	0.400	0.107	0.457	0.059	0.650
Problem Orientation Index	0.075	0.422	0.075	0.270	−0.100	0.451	0.072	0.500
Health Problem Index	0.012	0.892	0.096	0.090	−0.139	0.297	0.150	0.080
Behavior Complexity Index	0.233	0.012	0.155	0.000	0.062	0.610	0.158	0.060
Emotional Problem Index	0.561	0.000	0.289	0.000	0.253	0.049	0.150	0.130
General Social Support Index	0.058	0.533	0.061	0.420	−0.170	0.163	0.075	0.610
Training Activity Index	−0.576	0.000	0.304	0.000	−0.434	0.002	0.250	0.000
Recovery Environment Risk Index	−0.006	0.952	0.076	0.530	−0.083	0.541	0.055	0.970
Prior opiate use	0.420	0.000	0.209	0.000	0.173	0.201	0.086	0.180
Need for heroin treatment (self-reported)	0.636	0.000	0.290	0.000	0.614	0.000	0.280	0.000
Seizures/current withdrawal symptoms	0.010	0.915	0.004	0.890	0.026	0.835	0.010	0.830
Using daily	0.298	0.003	0.101	0.010	0.004	0.978	0.001	1.000
Using opioids[d]	0.278	0.002	0.136	0.000	0.167	0.195	0.082	0.160
Used in past two days	0.354	0.000	0.162	0.000	0.141	0.288	0.065	0.200
Substance use despite prior treatment	0.218	0.018	0.105	0.020	0.128	0.325	0.062	0.310
Acute health problems	−0.058	0.537	0.028	0.460	−0.159	0.252	0.076	0.230
High behavioral problems[a]	0.236	0.012	0.118	0.000	0.193	0.152	0.096	0.150
Days of victimization[c]	0.029	0.758	0.014	0.630	−0.020	0.883	0.010	0.840
High victimization	0.045	0.636	0.019	0.640	0.034	0.806	0.015	0.830
Current criminal justice involvement	0.260	0.008	0.100	0.010	0.129	0.338	0.050	0.360
Total arrests[c]	0.038	0.745	0.136	0.010	0.012	0.952	0.087	0.230
Mental distress	0.472	0.000	0.228	0.000	0.195	0.156	0.094	0.140
High resistance	−0.411	0.000	0.129	0.000	−0.273	0.063	0.086	0.050
Low motivation	0.005	0.959	0.002	0.980	−0.027	0.840	0.013	0.880
Low alc/drug use problem orientation	−0.023	0.807	0.011	0.790	0.103	0.436	0.050	0.430
First high/intoxicated under age 15	−0.186	0.036	0.063	0.010	−0.169	0.151	0.057	0.150
Needle use[c]	0.470	0.000	0.191	0.000	0.457	0.000	0.186	0.000
In school	−0.450	0.000	0.224	0.000	−0.331	0.013	0.165	0.000
Employed	0.326	0.000	0.163	0.000	0.004	0.974	0.002	1.000
Homeless/runaway[a]	0.132	0.151	0.059	0.200	0.098	0.453	0.044	0.460
Family hist. of substance use	−0.255	0.004	0.097	0.000	−0.228	0.056	0.087	0.080
Weekly family problems[c]	0.034	0.720	0.017	0.620	−0.150	0.267	0.075	0.240
Drunk/high most of day[d]	0.559	0.000	0.300	0.000	0.174	0.207	0.119	0.230
Tobacco Dependence Index[b,e]	0.775	0.000	0.304	0.000	0.085	0.525	0.071	0.750

Table A.7—Continued

Variable	Unweighted				Weighted			
	Effect Size	P-value	KS Statistic	KS P-value	Effect Size	P-value	KS Statistic	KS P-value
Health Distress Index[a]	0.102	0.271	0.043	0.700	0.235	0.082	0.091	0.300
Homicidal-Suicidal Thought Index	−0.283	0.004	0.110	0.000	−0.186	0.201	0.072	0.140
Lifetime detox admissions	0.277	0.001	0.136	0.000	0.244	0.013	0.105	0.080
Attended AA or other self-help	0.255	0.007	0.126	0.020	−0.055	0.669	0.027	0.660
Last grade completed in school	0.189	0.038	0.113	0.030	−0.036	0.778	0.093	0.270
Mention of alc as treatment need	−0.274	0.005	0.119	0.000	−0.185	0.198	0.081	0.170
Mention of marijuana as treatment need	0.005	0.954	0.003	0.960	−0.210	0.088	0.103	0.080
Mention of cocaine as treatment need	0.167	0.063	0.060	0.000	0.202	0.071	0.072	0.080
Mention of opiates as treatment need	0.677	0.000	0.316	0.000	0.656	0.000	0.306	0.000
Mention of amph's as treatment need	NA	0.000	0.111	0.000	NA	0.000	0.094	0.000
Mention of other drugs as treatment need	−0.091	0.354	0.020	0.330	−0.136	0.402	0.030	0.370
Controlled environment[c]	0.087	0.383	0.167	0.000	0.088	0.572	0.137	0.200
Currently in alc/drug treatment	−0.111	0.249	0.040	0.210	−0.214	0.167	0.078	0.160
Gender								
Male	0.292	0.849	0.120	0.000	0.194	NA	0.080	0.180
Female	−0.292	NA	0.120	0.000	−0.194	0.897	0.080	0.180
Race								
Am. Indian	−1.903	0.939	0.264	0.000	−0.420	NA	0.058	0.010
Black	0.600	NA	0.270	0.000	0.452	0.995	0.203	0.000
White	0.597	NA	0.284	0.000	−0.110	NA	0.052	0.350
Mexican	NA	NA	0.175	0.000	NA	NA	0.050	0.000
Other race	−0.552	NA	0.115	0.000	−0.203	NA	0.042	0.190
Substance most likes								
Alcohol	−0.207	NA	0.063	0.050	−0.009	NA	0.003	0.970
Cannabis	−0.244	NA	0.121	0.010	−0.396	NA	0.196	0.000
Crack or cocaine	−0.046	NA	0.008	0.530	−0.009	NA	0.002	0.980
Opiates	0.549	0.999	0.233	0.000	0.526	1.000	0.223	0.000
Hallucinogens	0.113	NA	0.025	0.160	0.073	NA	0.016	0.620
Amphetamines	NA	NA	0.066	0.000	NA	NA	0.043	0.000
Other substance	−0.003	NA	0.000	0.840	0.046	NA	0.004	0.660
Current living status								
House/apt	−0.558	NA	0.278	0.000	−0.555	0.974	0.277	0.000
Friend/relative	0.022	NA	0.006	0.830	0.066	NA	0.018	0.500
Jail/correctional	0.647	0.953	0.300	0.000	0.535	NA	0.248	0.000
Other status	−0.108	NA	0.028	0.300	0.041	NA	0.011	0.730

Table A.7—Continued

	N	Effective Sample Size	Average Effect Size	Max Effect Size	Average KS Statistic	Max KS Statistic	KS P-value
Unweighted	XXX[e]	XXX[e]	0.279	1.903	0.134	0.316	0.000
Weighted	XXX[e]	86.628	0.179	0.656	0.100	0.306	0.000

[a] Past year.

[b] Past month.

[c] Past 90 days.

[d] Weekly.

[e] Sample sizes censored in these tables to preserve program anonymity. For available sample sizes, see Table A.1.

Table A.8
Baseline Covariate Differences Between Program and Comparison Groups Before and After Weighting: Site E

	Unweighted				Weighted			
Variable	Effect Size	P-value	KS Statistic	KS P-value	Effect Size	P-value	KS Statistic	KS P-value
Age	−0.486	0.000	0.212	0.000	−0.206	0.134	0.103	0.180
Times received treatment for drug/alc	−0.094	0.258	0.198	0.000	0.014	0.865	0.093	0.120
Prior treatment psychological problems	−0.344	0.000	0.163	0.000	−0.220	0.076	0.104	0.050
No. people lived with[a]	0.079	0.343	0.030	0.930	0.109	0.247	0.064	0.660
Substance Dependence Index[a]	−0.121	0.179	0.054	0.490	−0.084	0.452	0.057	0.710
Substance Dependence Index[b]	−0.392	0.000	0.194	0.000	−0.247	0.043	0.130	0.070
Drug Crime Index, minus L3t	0.406	0.000	0.171	0.000	0.291	0.013	0.128	0.060
Living Risk Index	0.330	0.000	0.158	0.000	0.215	0.067	0.111	0.170
Vocational Risk Index	0.511	0.000	0.254	0.000	0.164	0.165	0.116	0.120
Social Risk Index	0.369	0.000	0.233	0.000	0.123	0.288	0.091	0.400
Needle Frequency Index	−0.742	0.000	0.081	0.000	−0.199	0.191	0.045	0.170
Needle Problem Index	−0.876	0.000	0.078	0.000	−0.429	0.044	0.043	0.130
Sex Protection Ratio	−0.055	0.546	0.047	0.590	0.035	0.776	0.046	0.870
Controlled Environment Index	0.525	0.000	0.302	0.000	0.365	0.001	0.200	0.020
General Satisfaction Index	−0.040	0.667	0.028	0.980	0.018	0.880	0.034	1.000
Mental Health Treatment Index	−0.601	0.000	0.113	0.000	−0.395	0.028	0.077	0.110
Criminal Justice System Index	0.888	0.000	0.363	0.000	0.478	0.000	0.233	0.000
Training Problem Index	0.133	0.147	0.079	0.190	−0.051	0.658	0.046	0.850
Substance Abuse Treatment Index	−0.380	0.001	0.191	0.000	−0.207	0.128	0.097	0.120
Substance Problem Index[a]	0.058	0.526	0.043	0.790	0.052	0.661	0.069	0.650
Substance Problem Index[b]	−0.322	0.001	0.143	0.010	−0.242	0.041	0.120	0.090
Physical Health Treatment Index	0.128	0.135	0.115	0.010	0.074	0.432	0.041	0.840

Table A.8—Continued

Variable	Unweighted				Weighted			
	Effect Size	P-value	KS Statistic	KS P-value	Effect Size	P-value	KS Statistic	KS P-value
Internal Mental Distress Index	0.299	0.001	0.155	0.000	0.190	0.099	0.101	0.330
Environmental Risk Index	0.683	0.000	0.323	0.000	0.273	0.027	0.125	0.050
General Victimization Index	0.392	0.000	0.200	0.000	0.275	0.017	0.173	0.020
Personal Sources of Stress Index	−0.041	0.661	0.027	0.910	−0.147	0.235	0.051	0.730
Other Sources of Stress Index	0.043	0.637	0.044	0.590	−0.040	0.733	0.027	0.990
Employment Problem Index	−0.075	0.419	0.038	0.760	−0.078	0.507	0.084	0.310
Employment Activity Index	0.001	0.995	0.047	0.770	0.025	0.839	0.036	0.990
Crime Violence Index	0.368	0.000	0.193	0.000	0.103	0.377	0.084	0.420
Illegal Activities Index	0.125	0.207	0.135	0.010	−0.096	0.424	0.118	0.120
Substance Frequency Index	−0.235	0.016	0.125	0.030	−0.270	0.023	0.131	0.200
Current Withdrawal Index	−0.383	0.000	0.222	0.000	−0.228	0.076	0.138	0.070
Treatment Resistance Index	−0.160	0.083	0.068	0.180	−0.044	0.707	0.035	0.850
Treatment Motivation Index	−0.181	0.045	0.063	0.270	−0.080	0.472	0.036	0.900
Self-Efficacy Index	0.008	0.932	0.037	0.780	−0.042	0.738	0.027	0.960
Problem Orientation Index	−0.078	0.397	0.053	0.460	−0.008	0.950	0.052	0.640
Health Problem Index	0.294	0.001	0.206	0.000	0.147	0.179	0.082	0.550
Behavior Complexity Index	0.156	0.099	0.099	0.050	0.032	0.791	0.080	0.630
Emotional Problem Index	−0.151	0.118	0.089	0.280	−0.208	0.076	0.120	0.250
General Social Support Index	0.411	0.000	0.164	0.000	0.206	0.135	0.086	0.370
Training Activity Index	0.094	0.307	0.067	0.630	−0.075	0.523	0.058	0.940
Recovery Environment Risk Index	0.337	0.000	0.172	0.000	0.034	0.768	0.071	0.810
Prior opiate use	−0.108	0.240	0.051	0.230	−0.219	0.081	0.104	0.080
Need for heroin treatment (self-reported)	−1.311	0.000	0.101	0.000	−0.589	0.009	0.046	0.030
Seizures/current withdrawal symptoms	−0.140	0.139	0.049	0.200	−0.105	0.386	0.037	0.420
Using daily	−0.097	0.282	0.041	0.180	−0.149	0.205	0.063	0.190
Using opioids[d]	0.219	0.014	0.106	0.010	0.162	0.176	0.078	0.150
Used in past two days	−0.195	0.043	0.066	0.060	−0.149	0.270	0.050	0.230
Substance use despite prior treatment	−0.756	0.000	0.241	0.000	−0.366	0.010	0.117	0.010
Acute health problems	0.220	0.015	0.109	0.000	0.103	0.393	0.051	0.440
High behavioral problems[a]	0.052	0.567	0.026	0.560	0.027	0.823	0.014	0.760
Days of victimization[c]	−0.038	0.675	0.018	0.700	−0.100	0.417	0.048	0.380
High victimization	0.052	0.572	0.023	0.690	0.043	0.729	0.019	0.680
Current criminal justice involvement	0.758	0.000	0.224	0.000	0.464	0.002	0.137	0.000
Total arrests[c]	0.113	0.247	0.156	0.000	0.081	0.483	0.059	0.480
Mental distress	−0.017	0.853	0.008	0.890	−0.005	0.968	0.002	0.950
High resistance	−0.118	0.208	0.045	0.190	−0.015	0.897	0.006	0.900
Low motivation	0.120	0.185	0.058	0.200	0.038	0.748	0.019	0.700

Table A.8—Continued

Variable	Unweighted				Weighted			
	Effect Size	P-value	KS Statistic	KS P-value	Effect Size	P-value	KS Statistic	KS P-value
Low alc/drug use problem orientation	0.044	0.628	0.022	0.630	−0.006	0.962	0.003	0.980
First high/intoxicated under age 15	0.357	0.001	0.067	0.000	0.107	0.419	0.020	0.410
Needle use[c]	−0.391	0.001	0.060	0.010	−0.054	0.603	0.008	0.770
In school	0.063	0.495	0.028	0.560	−0.093	0.417	0.042	0.390
Employed	−0.008	0.934	0.004	0.950	0.021	0.864	0.010	0.830
Homeless/runaway[a]	0.034	0.713	0.014	0.760	0.070	0.543	0.030	0.590
Family hist. of substance use	0.172	0.080	0.045	0.190	0.134	0.289	0.035	0.360
Weekly family problems[c]	0.148	0.105	0.074	0.100	−0.074	0.538	0.037	0.540
Drunk/high most of day[d]	−0.043	0.644	0.116	0.030	−0.194	0.101	0.153	0.020
Tobacco Dependence Index[b,e]	−0.134	0.151	0.180	0.000	−0.223	0.067	0.150	0.070
Health Distress Index[a]	−0.082	0.369	0.043	0.590	−0.039	0.752	0.028	0.950
Homicidal-Suicidal Thought Index	−0.076	0.414	0.032	0.450	−0.015	0.899	0.007	0.920
Lifetime detox admissions	−0.153	0.113	0.068	0.010	−0.068	0.561	0.025	0.560
Attended AA or other self-help	−0.367	0.000	0.177	0.000	−0.324	0.009	0.156	0.000
Last grade completed in school	−0.597	0.000	0.231	0.000	−0.368	0.002	0.168	0.010
Mention of alc as treatment need	−0.333	0.001	0.142	0.000	−0.163	0.202	0.070	0.250
Mention of marijuana as treatment need	−0.042	0.644	0.021	0.640	0.028	0.821	0.014	0.830
Mention of cocaine as treatment need	0.322	0.000	0.129	0.000	0.255	0.013	0.102	0.030
Mention of opiates as treatment need	−1.432	0.000	0.111	0.000	−0.660	0.004	0.051	0.010
Mention of amph's as treatment need	0.184	0.032	0.061	0.040	−0.047	0.737	0.015	0.670
Mention of other drugs as treatment need	0.227	0.007	0.074	0.000	0.049	0.673	0.016	0.710
Controlled environment[c]	0.463	0.000	0.293	0.000	0.357	0.001	0.206	0.010
Currently in alc/drug treatment	0.021	0.820	0.008	0.910	0.047	0.691	0.019	0.700
Gender								
Male	0.011	0.994	0.005	0.880	−0.021	0.988	0.010	0.860
Female	−0.011	NA	0.005	0.880	0.021	NA	0.010	0.860
Race								
Am. Indian	−2.588	0.952	0.282	0.000	−0.672	0.988	0.073	0.000
Black	−0.875	NA	0.095	0.000	−0.510	NA	0.056	0.020
White	−0.146	NA	0.071	0.140	−0.331	NA	0.162	0.010
Mexican	0.775	NA	0.380	0.000	0.645	NA	0.316	0.000
Other race	0.178	NA	0.069	0.050	−0.067	NA	0.026	0.620
Substance most likes								
Alcohol	−0.259	NA	0.077	0.020	−0.117	NA	0.035	0.320
Cannabis	−0.022	NA	0.011	0.780	−0.054	NA	0.026	0.590

Table A.8—Continued

Variable	Unweighted				Weighted			
	Effect Size	P-value	KS Statistic	KS P-value	Effect Size	P-value	KS Statistic	KS P-value
Crack or cocaine	0.292	NA	0.088	0.000	0.274	NA	0.083	0.000
Opiates	−1.009	1.000	0.078	0.000	−0.339	1.000	0.026	0.070
Hallucinogens	0.126	NA	0.029	0.060	0.039	NA	0.009	0.690
Amphetamines	0.126	NA	0.033	0.100	−0.084	NA	0.022	0.560
Other substance	0.118	NA	0.016	0.020	0.125	NA	0.017	0.170
Current living status								
House/apt	0.512	NA	0.174	0.000	0.197	NA	0.067	0.100
Friend/relative	−0.044	NA	0.011	0.630	−0.015	NA	0.004	0.920
Jail/correctional	−1.522	0.987	0.118	0.000	−0.955	0.995	0.074	0.000
Other status	−0.189	NA	0.045	0.080	0.046	NA	0.011	0.690

	N	Effective Sample Size	Average Effect Size	Max Effect Size	Average KS Statistic	Max KS Statistic	KS P-value
Unweighted	XXX[e]	XXX[e]	0.312	2.588	0.107	0.380	0.000
Weighted	XXX[e]	113.627	0.173	0.955	0.070	0.316	0.000

[a] Past year.

[b] Past month.

[c] Past 90 days.

[d] Weekly.

[e] Sample sizes censored in these tables to preserve program anonymity. For available sample sizes, see Table A.1.

Table A.9
Baseline Covariate Differences Between Program and Comparison Groups Before and After Weighting: Site F

Variable	Unweighted				Weighted			
	Effect Size	P-value	KS Statistic	KS P-value	Effect Size	P-value	KS Statistic	KS P-value
Age	0.000	0.996	0.074	0.190	0.241	0.129	0.221	0.150
Times received treatment for drug/alc	−0.156	0.169	0.054	0.390	0.084	0.615	0.055	0.820
Prior treatment psychological problems	−0.743	0.000	0.305	0.000	−0.368	0.163	0.151	0.130
No. people lived with[a]	0.141	0.235	0.197	0.000	−0.052	0.858	0.106	0.800
Substance Dependence Index[a]	−0.139	0.160	0.062	0.520	−0.044	0.803	0.128	0.620
Substance Dependence Index[b]	−0.583	0.000	0.185	0.000	−0.365	0.123	0.154	0.400
Drug Crime Index, minus L3t	−0.813	0.000	0.365	0.000	−0.433	0.100	0.183	0.160
Living Risk Index	−0.297	0.006	0.116	0.020	−0.045	0.829	0.098	0.870
Vocational Risk Index	−0.322	0.003	0.225	0.000	0.093	0.753	0.123	0.730
Social Risk Index	−0.594	0.000	0.286	0.000	−0.487	0.055	0.207	0.140
Needle Frequency Index	−1.384	0.000	0.074	0.030	−1.290	0.331	0.065	0.370
Needle Problem Index	−0.778	0.000	0.080	0.000	−0.795	0.318	0.062	0.090
Sex Protection Ratio	0.584	0.000	0.278	0.000	0.190	0.394	0.135	0.190

Table A.9—Continued

Variable	Unweighted				Weighted			
	Effect Size	P-value	KS Statistic	KS P-value	Effect Size	P-value	KS Statistic	KS P-value
Controlled Environment Index	−0.117	0.238	0.158	0.000	−0.178	0.365	0.252	0.080
General Satisfaction Index	0.580	0.000	0.252	0.000	0.155	0.598	0.198	0.310
Mental Health Treatment Index	−1.925	0.000	0.171	0.000	−1.710	0.073	0.156	0.040
Criminal Justice System Index	−0.078	0.437	0.053	0.540	0.069	0.743	0.083	0.830
Training Problem Index	−0.231	0.025	0.148	0.020	−0.233	0.296	0.160	0.370
Substance Abuse Treatment Index	0.135	0.156	0.082	0.220	0.177	0.241	0.199	0.110
Substance Problem Index[a]	−0.215	0.030	0.116	0.030	0.012	0.958	0.070	1.000
Substance Problem Index[b]	−0.693	0.000	0.251	0.000	−0.362	0.114	0.186	0.310
Physical Health Treatment Index	−0.891	0.000	0.231	0.000	−0.439	0.136	0.146	0.230
Internal Mental Distress Index	−0.364	0.000	0.212	0.000	−0.130	0.399	0.247	0.130
Environmental Risk Index	−0.581	0.000	0.262	0.000	−0.203	0.406	0.134	0.670
General Victimization Index	−0.382	0.000	0.119	0.040	−0.183	0.457	0.084	0.940
Personal Sources of Stress Index	−0.354	0.001	0.190	0.010	−0.349	0.087	0.184	0.200
Other Sources of Stress Index	−0.476	0.000	0.198	0.000	−0.306	0.197	0.148	0.300
Employment Problem Index	−0.678	0.000	0.248	0.000	−0.435	0.106	0.128	0.340
Employment Activity Index	−0.508	0.000	0.236	0.000	−0.318	0.174	0.182	0.140
Crime Violence Index	−1.074	0.000	0.380	0.000	−0.400	0.048	0.286	0.030
Illegal Activities Index	−0.836	0.000	0.383	0.000	−0.667	0.000	0.354	0.020
Substance Frequency Index	−1.118	0.000	0.460	0.000	−0.613	0.017	0.338	0.000
Current Withdrawal Index	0.203	0.043	0.170	0.000	0.025	0.925	0.148	0.560
Treatment Resistance Index	0.111	0.274	0.054	0.440	0.222	0.200	0.179	0.230
Treatment Motivation Index	0.232	0.035	0.114	0.010	0.088	0.731	0.093	0.650
Self-Efficacy Index	−0.011	0.915	0.032	0.780	−0.064	0.713	0.043	0.970
Problem Orientation Index	−0.196	0.053	0.108	0.030	0.203	0.348	0.116	0.570
Health Problem Index	−1.259	0.000	0.440	0.000	−0.550	0.013	0.312	0.010
Behavior Complexity Index	−0.541	0.000	0.209	0.000	−0.330	0.065	0.188	0.310
Emotional Problem Index	−0.903	0.000	0.354	0.000	−0.595	0.010	0.319	0.030
General Social Support Index	−0.607	0.000	0.279	0.000	−0.200	0.599	0.265	0.010
Training Activity Index	−0.072	0.457	0.148	0.030	−0.145	0.442	0.156	0.620
Recovery Environment Risk Index	−1.680	0.000	0.547	0.000	−0.914	0.011	0.346	0.040
Prior opiate use	−0.912	0.000	0.312	0.000	−0.462	0.099	0.158	0.050
Need for heroin treatment (self-reported)	−1.018	0.000	0.090	0.000	−0.916	0.186	0.081	0.010
Seizures/current withdrawal symptoms	0.082	0.407	0.033	0.360	−0.156	0.553	0.063	0.520
Using daily	−0.478	0.000	0.233	0.000	−0.396	0.023	0.193	0.050
Using opioids[d]	−2.796	0.000	0.350	0.000	−1.731	0.029	0.216	0.000

Table A.9—Continued

Variable	Unweighted				Weighted			
	Effect Size	P-value	KS Statistic	KS P-value	Effect Size	P-value	KS Statistic	KS P-value
Used in past two days	−0.473	0.000	0.128	0.000	−0.164	0.625	0.044	0.430
Substance use despite prior treatment	−0.075	0.459	0.033	0.440	−0.058	0.810	0.026	0.830
Acute health problems	−0.862	0.000	0.295	0.000	−0.328	0.155	0.112	0.170
High behavioral problems[a]	−0.273	0.008	0.126	0.000	0.017	0.936	0.008	0.970
Days of victimization[c]	−0.542	0.000	0.216	0.000	−0.392	0.127	0.156	0.110
High victimization	−0.172	0.082	0.081	0.080	−0.061	0.803	0.029	0.800
Current criminal justice involvement	0.108	0.290	0.045	0.370	0.210	0.426	0.087	0.360
Total arrests[c]	0.058	0.527	0.206	0.000	0.086	0.422	0.226	0.060
Mental distress	−0.484	0.000	0.219	0.000	0.020	0.931	0.009	0.930
High resistance	0.092	0.351	0.039	0.310	0.264	0.072	0.112	0.240
Low motivation	−0.252	0.015	0.109	0.000	0.023	0.907	0.010	0.970
Low alc/drug use problem orientation	0.169	0.091	0.084	0.060	−0.231	0.288	0.115	0.360
First high/intoxicated under age 15	−0.079	0.420	0.024	0.330	−0.108	0.469	0.033	0.700
Needle use[c]	−0.523	0.000	0.065	0.010	−0.408	0.378	0.051	0.110
In school	−0.234	0.018	0.114	0.010	−0.224	0.261	0.109	0.390
Employed	−0.519	0.000	0.213	0.000	−0.370	0.142	0.152	0.110
Homeless/runaway[a]	−0.395	0.000	0.132	0.000	−0.504	0.136	0.168	0.040
Family hist. of substance use	0.005	0.960	0.002	0.950	0.096	0.780	0.029	0.680
Weekly family problems[c]	−1.063	0.000	0.388	0.000	−0.657	0.023	0.240	0.000
Drunk/high most of day[d]	−1.225	0.000	0.464	0.000	−0.692	0.072	0.318	0.020
Tobacco Dependence Index[b,e]	−0.994	0.000	0.458	0.000	−0.795	0.000	0.382	0.000
Health Distress Index[a]	−0.040	0.688	0.020	0.970	−0.032	0.869	0.048	0.920
Homicidal-Suicidal Thought Index	−0.078	0.441	0.033	0.440	−0.130	0.623	0.055	0.580
Lifetime detox admissions	−0.011	0.918	0.027	0.700	0.072	0.757	0.064	0.500
Attended AA or other self-help	0.033	0.743	0.016	0.740	−0.065	0.778	0.033	0.800
Last grade completed in school	−0.025	0.806	0.064	0.330	0.172	0.302	0.154	0.300
Mention of alc as treatment need	0.768	0.000	0.370	0.000	0.367	0.131	0.176	0.110
Mention of marijuana as treatment need	0.227	0.026	0.106	0.040	−0.109	0.575	0.051	0.680
Mention of cocaine as treatment need	−1.404	0.000	0.125	0.000	−1.304	0.076	0.116	0.000
Mention of opiates as treatment need	−1.115	0.000	0.099	0.000	−0.917	0.185	0.081	0.010
Mention of amph's as treatment need	−0.677	0.000	0.085	0.000	−0.182	0.364	0.023	0.510
Mention of other drugs as treatment need	−0.850	0.000	0.075	0.000	−0.375	0.307	0.033	0.160
Controlled environment[c]	0.015	0.875	0.127	0.070	−0.003	0.986	0.239	0.140

Table A.9—Continued

Variable	Unweighted				Weighted			
	Effect Size	P-value	KS Statistic	KS P-value	Effect Size	P-value	KS Statistic	KS P-value
Currently in alc/drug treatment	−0.228	0.030	0.076	0.030	−0.199	0.373	0.066	0.430
Gender								
Male	−0.118	NA	0.056	0.220	0.192	0.895	0.091	0.400
Female	0.118	0.932	0.056	0.230	−0.192	NA	0.091	0.400
Race								
Am. Indian	4.039	0.779	0.925	0.000	1.926	0.974	0.441	0.000
Black	NA	NA	0.103	0.000	NA	NA	0.034	0.080
White	NA	NA	0.562	0.000	NA	NA	0.027	0.090
Mexican	NA	NA	0.165	0.000	NA	NA	0.029	0.060
Other race	−0.420	NA	0.096	0.000	−1.536	NA	0.352	0.000
Substance most likes								
Alcohol	0.194	NA	0.080	0.010	0.310	1.000	0.127	0.160
Cannabis	0.336	1.000	0.142	0.000	−0.015	NA	0.006	0.930
Crack or cocaine	NA	NA	0.049	0.030	NA	NA	0.012	0.070
Opiates	NA	NA	0.079	0.000	NA	NA	0.064	0.030
Hallucinogens	NA	NA	0.043	0.020	NA	NA	0.025	0.090
Amphetamines	−0.335	NA	0.042	0.140	−0.157	NA	0.020	0.530
Other substance	NA	NA	0.009	0.350	NA	NA	0.000	0.000
Current living status								
House/apt	−0.163	NA	0.076	0.060	−0.282	NA	0.131	0.150
Friend/relative	−0.158	NA	0.034	0.210	−0.488	NA	0.104	0.010
Jail/correctional	−0.428	NA	0.075	0.030	0.105	NA	0.018	0.750
Other status	0.434	0.982	0.185	0.000	0.509	0.968	0.217	0.040

	N	Effective Sample Size	Average Effect Size	Max Effect Size	Average KS Statistic	Max KS Statistic	KS P-value
Unweighted	XXX[e]	XXX[e]	0.534	4.039	0.174	0.925	0.000
Weighted	XXX[e]	22.117	0.363	1.926	0.134	0.441	0.010

[a] Past year.

[b] Past month.

[c] Past 90 days.

[d] Weekly.

[e] Sample sizes censored in these tables to preserve program anonymity. For available sample sizes, see Table A.1.

Table A.10
Baseline Covariate Differences Between Program and Comparison Groups Before and After Weighting: Site G

Variable	Unweighted				Weighted			
	Effect Size	P-value	KS Statistic	KS P-value	Effect Size	P-value	KS Statistic	KS P-value
Age	−0.107	0.267	0.061	0.300	−0.047	0.689	0.063	0.660
Times received treatment for drug/alc	−0.177	0.092	0.095	0.060	−0.086	0.415	0.054	0.740
Prior treatment psychological problems	0.638	0.000	0.298	0.000	0.374	0.012	0.175	0.010
No. people lived with[a]	−0.223	0.035	0.111	0.040	−0.021	0.854	0.063	0.700
Substance Dependence Index[a]	−0.018	0.852	0.054	0.590	−0.051	0.665	0.061	0.750
Substance Dependence Index[b]	0.521	0.000	0.281	0.000	0.135	0.295	0.072	0.750
Drug Crime Index, minus L3t	−0.102	0.297	0.087	0.080	0.036	0.796	0.054	0.690
Living Risk Index	−0.053	0.593	0.062	0.460	0.037	0.777	0.042	0.940
Vocational Risk Index	0.334	0.001	0.183	0.000	−0.047	0.700	0.077	0.790
Social Risk Index	−0.036	0.712	0.059	0.620	−0.184	0.194	0.128	0.250
Needle Frequency Index	−1.141	0.000	0.092	0.000	−0.362	0.018	0.042	0.250
Needle Problem Index	−0.409	0.001	0.063	0.020	−0.092	0.391	0.018	0.800
Sex Protection Ratio	0.059	0.532	0.053	0.580	−0.081	0.521	0.044	0.870
Controlled Environment Index	−1.158	0.000	0.343	0.000	−0.302	0.022	0.143	0.100
General Satisfaction Index	−0.314	0.001	0.174	0.000	−0.180	0.217	0.134	0.100
Mental Health Treatment Index	0.419	0.000	0.252	0.000	0.221	0.056	0.130	0.080
Criminal Justice System Index	−1.064	0.000	0.446	0.000	−0.404	0.007	0.182	0.020
Training Problem Index	0.599	0.000	0.214	0.000	0.117	0.340	0.070	0.640
Substance Abuse Treatment Index	0.126	0.165	0.113	0.050	0.102	0.374	0.137	0.110
Substance Problem Index[a]	−0.116	0.228	0.096	0.060	−0.127	0.279	0.110	0.330
Substance Problem Index[b]	0.628	0.000	0.297	0.000	0.187	0.149	0.111	0.340
Physical Health Treatment Index	0.098	0.396	0.187	0.000	−0.083	0.643	0.087	0.410
Internal Mental Distress Index	0.139	0.154	0.111	0.050	0.019	0.897	0.042	0.990
Environmental Risk Index	0.150	0.126	0.082	0.330	−0.108	0.403	0.101	0.570
General Victimization Index	−0.055	0.574	0.081	0.270	−0.134	0.398	0.094	0.420
Personal Sources of Stress Index	0.388	0.000	0.150	0.000	0.310	0.020	0.103	0.240
Other Sources of Stress Index	0.409	0.000	0.241	0.000	0.175	0.170	0.096	0.350
Employment Problem Index	−0.123	0.205	0.076	0.230	−0.137	0.273	0.114	0.220
Employment Activity Index	0.019	0.846	0.068	0.350	−0.151	0.294	0.091	0.480
Crime Violence Index	−0.072	0.476	0.136	0.010	−0.110	0.396	0.126	0.200
Illegal Activities Index	0.332	0.001	0.229	0.000	0.130	0.339	0.094	0.610
Substance Frequency Index	0.349	0.000	0.204	0.000	0.070	0.596	0.070	0.940

Table A.10—Continued

Variable	Unweighted				Weighted			
	Effect Size	P-value	KS Statistic	KS P-value	Effect Size	P-value	KS Statistic	KS P-value
Current Withdrawal Index	0.127	0.185	0.146	0.000	−0.049	0.756	0.076	0.760
Treatment Resistance Index	0.400	0.000	0.145	0.000	0.222	0.115	0.105	0.180
Treatment Motivation Index	−0.010	0.909	0.071	0.220	0.081	0.477	0.077	0.520
Self-Efficacy Index	−0.140	0.132	0.058	0.400	−0.020	0.892	0.026	1.000
Problem Orientation Index	0.175	0.066	0.080	0.130	0.133	0.327	0.060	0.740
Health Problem Index	0.358	0.000	0.261	0.000	0.065	0.661	0.109	0.390
Behavior Complexity Index	0.168	0.102	0.111	0.090	0.031	0.821	0.055	0.930
Emotional Problem Index	0.185	0.056	0.158	0.000	−0.114	0.402	0.095	0.700
General Social Support Index	0.152	0.117	0.080	0.170	−0.082	0.528	0.064	0.680
Training Activity Index	0.857	0.000	0.324	0.000	0.075	0.561	0.110	0.470
Recovery Environment Risk Index	0.624	0.000	0.302	0.000	0.285	0.016	0.133	0.220
Prior opiate use	0.239	0.011	0.119	0.030	0.067	0.638	0.034	0.670
Need for heroin treatment (self-reported)	NA	0.000	0.106	0.000	NA	0.000	0.042	0.010
Seizures/current withdrawal symptoms	0.049	0.603	0.019	0.460	0.092	0.448	0.036	0.480
Using daily	0.510	0.000	0.149	0.000	0.039	0.731	0.011	0.860
Using opioids[d]	0.125	0.181	0.059	0.130	0.107	0.398	0.051	0.480
Used in past two days	0.049	0.603	0.019	0.650	−0.028	0.827	0.011	0.890
Substance use despite prior treatment	0.365	0.000	0.180	0.000	0.223	0.145	0.110	0.100
Acute health problems	0.346	0.000	0.173	0.000	0.101	0.488	0.051	0.480
High behavioral problems[a]	−0.073	0.444	0.035	0.390	−0.027	0.843	0.013	0.760
Days of victimization[c]	0.396	0.000	0.198	0.000	0.102	0.484	0.051	0.440
High victimization	0.065	0.497	0.028	0.600	0.000	1.000	0.000	1.000
Current criminal justice involvement	−0.767	0.000	0.382	0.000	−0.294	0.054	0.147	0.030
Total arrests[c]	−0.321	0.005	0.123	0.020	−0.073	0.544	0.023	0.940
Mental distress	−0.058	0.539	0.029	0.600	−0.138	0.335	0.068	0.310
High resistance	0.311	0.001	0.145	0.000	0.116	0.432	0.054	0.350
Low motivation	0.067	0.477	0.032	0.490	−0.107	0.484	0.051	0.500
Low alc/drug use problem orientation	−0.185	0.054	0.087	0.070	−0.119	0.398	0.056	0.430
First high/intoxicated under age 15	0.053	0.585	0.014	0.590	0.066	0.664	0.017	0.710
Needle use[c]	−0.625	0.000	0.072	0.000	−0.227	0.073	0.026	0.250
In school	1.196	0.000	0.299	0.000	0.250	0.042	0.063	0.090
Employed	0.056	0.554	0.027	0.550	−0.141	0.328	0.069	0.320
Homeless/runaway[a]	0.094	0.312	0.042	0.300	−0.034	0.828	0.015	0.830
Family hist. of substance use	0.199	0.052	0.050	0.070	0.196	0.193	0.049	0.220
Weekly family problems[c]	0.522	0.000	0.249	0.000	0.162	0.249	0.077	0.340
Drunk/high most of day[d]	0.269	0.004	0.153	0.000	−0.003	0.981	0.070	0.920

Table A.10—Continued

Variable	Unweighted				Weighted			
	Effect Size	P-value	KS Statistic	KS P-value	Effect Size	P-value	KS Statistic	KS P-value
Tobacco Dependence Index[b,e]	0.299	0.002	0.209	0.000	−0.086	0.503	0.069	0.880
Health Distress Index[a]	0.018	0.856	0.035	0.720	0.073	0.595	0.056	0.690
Homicidal-Suicidal Thought Index	0.359	0.000	0.176	0.000	0.282	0.023	0.138	0.040
Lifetime detox admissions	−1.227	0.000	0.090	0.000	−0.924	0.028	0.064	0.080
Attended AA or other self-help	0.094	0.320	0.047	0.330	0.105	0.461	0.052	0.420
Last grade completed in school	0.437	0.000	0.195	0.000	0.083	0.565	0.052	0.690
Mention of alc as treatment need	−0.120	0.209	0.055	0.240	−0.151	0.312	0.069	0.360
Mention of marijuana as treatment need	−0.149	0.113	0.074	0.060	−0.118	0.408	0.059	0.430
Mention of cocaine as treatment need	−0.447	0.000	0.088	0.000	−0.284	0.057	0.056	0.110
Mention of opiates as treatment need	NA	0.000	0.115	0.000	NA	0.002	0.068	0.000
Mention of amph's as treatment need	0.324	0.000	0.123	0.000	0.126	0.328	0.048	0.290
Mention of other drugs as treatment need	0.033	0.723	0.009	0.680	−0.138	0.364	0.036	0.350
Controlled environment[c]	−1.214	0.000	0.349	0.000	−0.348	0.011	0.145	0.070
Currently in alc/drug treatment	0.227	0.013	0.100	0.010	0.152	0.306	0.067	0.290
Gender								
Male	−0.160	0.907	0.077	0.100	0.109	0.939	0.052	0.470
Female	0.160	NA	0.077	0.100	−0.109	NA	0.052	0.470
Race								
Am. Indian	−1.558	0.980	0.252	0.000	−0.406	0.999	0.066	0.060
Black	−0.577	NA	0.081	0.000	−0.213	NA	0.030	0.160
White	0.605	NA	0.287	0.000	0.157	NA	0.075	0.360
Mexican	−0.333	NA	0.083	0.010	−0.137	NA	0.034	0.310
Other race	0.308	NA	0.129	0.000	0.131	NA	0.055	0.350
Substance most likes								
Alcohol	0.186	NA	0.075	0.030	0.133	NA	0.054	0.430
Cannabis	0.017	NA	0.008	0.850	−0.004	NA	0.002	1.000
Crack or cocaine	−0.523	1.000	0.043	0.010	−0.198	1.000	0.016	0.220
Opiates	NA	NA	0.083	0.000	NA	NA	0.023	0.070
Hallucinogens	−0.129	NA	0.018	0.350	−0.128	NA	0.018	0.460
Amphetamines	0.230	NA	0.069	0.000	0.048	NA	0.015	0.580
Other substance	NA	NA	0.009	0.190	NA	NA	0.010	0.220
Current living status								
House/apt	0.483	NA	0.165	0.000	−0.005	NA	0.002	0.940
Friend/relative	0.118	NA	0.036	0.140	0.220	NA	0.066	0.110
Jail/correctional	−1.377	0.981	0.112	0.000	−0.387	0.995	0.032	0.110
Other status	−0.543	NA	0.088	0.000	−0.203	NA	0.033	0.300

Table A.10—Continued

	N	Effective Sample Size	Average Effect Size	Max Effect Size	Average KS Statistic	Max KS Statistic	KS P-value
Unweighted	XXX[e]	XXX[e]	0.341	1.558	0.129	0.446	0.000
Weighted	XXX[e]	74.701	0.145	0.924	0.066	0.182	0.680

[a] Past year.

[b] Past month.

[c] Past 90 days.

[d] Weekly.

[e] Sample sizes censored in these tables to preserve program anonymity. For available sample sizes, see Table A.1.

Table A.11
Baseline Covariate Differences Between Program and Comparison Groups Before and After Weighting: Site H

	Unweighted				Weighted			
Variable	Effect Size	P-value	KS Statistic	KS P-value	Effect Size	P-value	KS Statistic	KS P-value
Age	0.412	0.000	0.166	0.000	0.231	0.068	0.101	0.140
Times received treatment for drug/alc	−0.185	0.102	0.057	0.250	0.072	0.556	0.077	0.270
Prior treatment psychological problems	−0.043	0.650	0.021	0.690	0.046	0.691	0.022	0.660
No. people lived with[a]	0.172	0.039	0.074	0.170	0.113	0.238	0.059	0.650
Substance Dependence Index[a]	−0.543	0.000	0.235	0.000	−0.152	0.194	0.067	0.590
Substance Dependence Index[b]	−0.313	0.003	0.105	0.040	−0.083	0.502	0.030	0.880
Drug Crime Index, minus L3t	−0.058	0.555	0.079	0.090	−0.005	0.968	0.025	0.820
Living Risk Index	−0.047	0.632	0.041	0.820	0.083	0.456	0.058	0.780
Vocational Risk Index	−0.243	0.011	0.129	0.010	−0.097	0.408	0.070	0.680
Social Risk Index	−0.086	0.375	0.072	0.350	0.134	0.245	0.113	0.210
Needle Frequency Index	0.001	0.991	0.032	0.100	0.059	0.496	0.013	0.690
Needle Problem Index	0.067	0.429	0.017	0.240	0.116	0.153	0.019	0.150
Sex Protection Ratio	0.025	0.794	0.061	0.310	0.043	0.732	0.059	0.560
Controlled Environment Index	−0.253	0.008	0.302	0.000	−0.056	0.655	0.109	0.060
General Satisfaction Index	0.390	0.000	0.169	0.000	0.209	0.083	0.113	0.120
Mental Health Treatment Index	−0.025	0.779	0.083	0.030	0.062	0.451	0.051	0.280
Criminal Justice System Index	−0.368	0.000	0.230	0.000	−0.065	0.598	0.078	0.350
Training Problem Index	0.049	0.596	0.045	0.680	0.029	0.792	0.066	0.660
Substance Abuse Treatment Index	−0.322	0.005	0.138	0.000	−0.043	0.667	0.043	0.510
Substance Problem Index[a]	−0.619	0.000	0.242	0.000	−0.229	0.049	0.114	0.230
Substance Problem Index[b]	−0.345	0.001	0.109	0.040	−0.132	0.299	0.059	0.630
Physical Health Treatment Index	0.076	0.351	0.111	0.010	0.078	0.375	0.037	0.750

Table A.11—Continued

Variable	Unweighted				Weighted			
	Effect Size	P-value	KS Statistic	KS P-value	Effect Size	P-value	KS Statistic	KS P-value
Internal Mental Distress Index	−0.588	0.000	0.288	0.000	−0.262	0.035	0.151	0.060
Environmental Risk Index	−0.209	0.036	0.115	0.040	0.039	0.740	0.048	0.990
General Victimization Index	−0.203	0.043	0.194	0.000	−0.022	0.851	0.097	0.240
Personal Sources of Stress Index	−0.200	0.039	0.096	0.080	−0.149	0.222	0.072	0.470
Other Sources of Stress Index	−0.550	0.000	0.222	0.000	−0.263	0.026	0.151	0.020
Employment Problem Index	0.304	0.001	0.165	0.000	0.167	0.155	0.090	0.260
Employment Activity Index	0.315	0.001	0.166	0.000	0.087	0.461	0.083	0.600
Crime Violence Index	0.453	0.000	0.234	0.000	0.376	0.003	0.190	0.000
Illegal Activities Index	0.101	0.315	0.105	0.070	0.056	0.654	0.079	0.570
Substance Frequency Index	−0.109	0.268	0.079	0.400	0.058	0.621	0.077	0.700
Current Withdrawal Index	−0.398	0.000	0.105	0.020	−0.143	0.228	0.051	0.560
Treatment Resistance Index	−0.307	0.002	0.113	0.010	−0.065	0.608	0.023	0.910
Treatment Motivation Index	−0.117	0.230	0.057	0.400	0.038	0.755	0.029	0.940
Self-Efficacy Index	0.485	0.000	0.157	0.000	0.180	0.158	0.063	0.370
Problem Orientation Index	−0.300	0.002	0.145	0.000	−0.087	0.455	0.051	0.390
Health Problem Index	−0.063	0.507	0.064	0.490	−0.092	0.435	0.068	0.660
Behavior Complexity Index	−0.260	0.011	0.149	0.000	−0.066	0.589	0.052	0.950
Emotional Problem Index	−0.076	0.429	0.084	0.310	−0.048	0.675	0.093	0.580
General Social Support Index	−0.166	0.072	0.074	0.240	−0.091	0.441	0.049	0.820
Training Activity Index	−0.241	0.009	0.140	0.040	−0.158	0.155	0.094	0.480
Recovery Environment Risk Index	−0.322	0.002	0.140	0.020	−0.052	0.666	0.053	0.950
Prior opiate use	−0.104	0.279	0.044	0.380	0.062	0.585	0.026	0.620
Need for heroin treatment (self-reported)	0.162	0.043	0.025	0.000	0.162	0.043	0.025	0.030
Seizures/current withdrawal symptoms	−0.500	0.000	0.079	0.000	−0.350	0.022	0.055	0.060
Using daily	−0.027	0.774	0.012	0.810	0.008	0.944	0.004	0.960
Using opioids[d]	−0.168	0.095	0.046	0.130	0.024	0.826	0.007	0.800
Used in past two days	0.144	0.116	0.062	0.120	0.167	0.134	0.072	0.110
Substance use despite prior treatment	0.078	0.397	0.031	0.410	0.194	0.069	0.077	0.170
Acute health problems	−0.115	0.226	0.054	0.240	−0.145	0.235	0.069	0.320
High behavioral problems[a]	−0.331	0.001	0.121	0.000	−0.057	0.643	0.021	0.600
Days of victimization[c]	−0.227	0.021	0.088	0.010	−0.149	0.229	0.058	0.280
High victimization	−0.134	0.154	0.067	0.180	−0.035	0.772	0.017	0.790
Current criminal justice involvement	−0.257	0.005	0.117	0.000	−0.068	0.567	0.031	0.530
Total arrests[c]	−0.480	0.000	0.186	0.000	−0.136	0.246	0.063	0.250
Mental distress	−0.138	0.149	0.062	0.190	−0.056	0.646	0.025	0.640
High resistance	−0.217	0.035	0.058	0.030	−0.067	0.620	0.018	0.430
Low motivation	0.113	0.233	0.055	0.230	−0.031	0.793	0.015	0.850

Table A.11—Continued

	Unweighted				Weighted			
Variable	Effect Size	P-value	KS Statistic	KS P-value	Effect Size	P-value	KS Statistic	KS P-value
Low alc/drug use problem orientation	0.082	0.385	0.039	0.430	−0.048	0.682	0.023	0.650
First high/intoxicated under age 15	−0.067	0.469	0.022	0.490	0.040	0.768	0.013	0.710
Needle use[c]	0.003	0.975	0.000	0.990	0.064	0.463	0.007	0.480
In school	−0.215	0.017	0.090	0.000	−0.188	0.080	0.079	0.080
Employed	0.289	0.002	0.143	0.000	0.063	0.600	0.031	0.690
Homeless/runaway[a]	−0.289	0.006	0.074	0.000	−0.102	0.383	0.026	0.390
Family hist. of substance use	−0.196	0.033	0.092	0.010	−0.096	0.431	0.045	0.410
Weekly family problems[c]	−0.210	0.031	0.088	0.030	−0.064	0.580	0.027	0.580
Drunk/high most of day[d]	−0.267	0.008	0.109	0.070	−0.056	0.656	0.042	0.930
Tobacco Dependence Index[b,e]	0.197	0.034	0.225	0.000	0.026	0.820	0.092	0.260
Health Distress Index[a]	−0.043	0.656	0.032	0.780	0.028	0.815	0.016	0.970
Homicidal-Suicidal Thought Index	−0.200	0.046	0.065	0.090	−0.080	0.495	0.026	0.650
Lifetime detox admissions	0.085	0.293	0.017	0.430	0.117	0.146	0.024	0.250
Attended AA or other self-help	−0.140	0.145	0.061	0.110	0.026	0.816	0.012	0.870
Last grade completed in school	0.473	0.000	0.238	0.000	0.187	0.101	0.091	0.210
Mention of alc as treatment need	−0.210	0.039	0.060	0.040	−0.096	0.419	0.027	0.480
Mention of marijuana as treatment need	0.039	0.680	0.019	0.650	−0.012	0.923	0.006	0.900
Mention of cocaine as treatment need	−0.150	0.146	0.029	0.220	−0.025	0.825	0.005	0.900
Mention of opiates as treatment need	0.085	0.321	0.012	0.210	0.062	0.511	0.008	0.550
Mention of amph's as treatment need	NA	0.000	0.047	0.010	NA	0.024	0.025	0.070
Mention of other drugs as treatment need	−0.169	0.120	0.023	0.170	−0.104	0.409	0.014	0.450
Controlled environment[c]	−0.234	0.016	0.296	0.000	−0.053	0.653	0.103	0.090
Currently in alc/drug treatment	−1.303	0.000	0.146	0.000	−0.656	0.001	0.074	0.000
Gender								
Male	0.290	NA	0.101	0.020	0.210	NA	0.073	0.110
Female	−0.290	0.856	0.101	0.020	−0.210	0.892	0.073	0.110
Race								
Am. Indian	−0.138	NA	0.011	0.340	0.051	NA	0.004	0.580
Black	0.303	NA	0.125	0.000	0.140	0.999	0.058	0.260
White	0.365	NA	0.165	0.000	0.015	NA	0.007	0.930
Mexican	NA	NA	0.156	0.000	NA	NA	0.058	0.000
Other race	−0.501	0.990	0.122	0.000	−0.042	NA	0.010	0.680
Substance most likes								
Alcohol	0.216	1.000	0.087	0.010	0.112	NA	0.045	0.290
Cannabis	−0.155	NA	0.071	0.010	−0.111	NA	0.051	0.310

Table A.11—Continued

Variable	Unweighted				Weighted			
	Effect Size	P-value	KS Statistic	KS P-value	Effect Size	P-value	KS Statistic	KS P-value
Crack or cocaine	0.026	NA	0.005	0.690	0.059	NA	0.010	0.530
Opiates	0.121	NA	0.017	0.020	0.098	NA	0.013	0.310
Hallucinogens	−0.106	NA	0.017	0.340	−0.109	NA	0.017	0.480
Amphetamines	NA	NA	0.037	0.030	NA	NA	0.016	0.120
Other substance	0.121	NA	0.017	0.020	0.113	1.000	0.015	0.290
Current living status								
House/apt	−0.058	NA	0.022	0.570	−0.055	NA	0.020	0.630
Friend/relative	0.252	0.991	0.094	0.000	0.182	0.996	0.068	0.100
Jail/correctional	NA	NA	0.050	0.010	NA	NA	0.034	0.020
Other status	NA	NA	0.022	0.070	NA	NA	0.013	0.130

	N	Effective Sample Size	Average Effect Size	Max Effect Size	Average KS Statistic	Max KS Statistic	KS P-value
Unweighted	XXX[e]	XXX[e]	0.226	1.303	0.097	0.302	0.000
Weighted	XXX[e]	126.111	0.106	0.656	0.050	0.190	0.150

[a] Past year.

[b] Past month.

[c] Past 90 days.

[d] Weekly.

[e] Sample sizes censored in these tables to preserve program anonymity. For available sample sizes, see Table A.1.

Table A.12
Baseline Covariate Differences Between Program and Comparison Groups Before and After Weighting: Site I

Variable	Unweighted				Weighted			
	Effect Size	P-value	KS Statistic	KS P-value	Effect Size	P-value	KS Statistic	KS P-value
Age	0.306	0.002	0.121	0.010	0.177	0.143	0.054	0.660
Times received treatment for drug/alc	−0.612	0.000	0.139	0.000	−0.248	0.079	0.072	0.320
Prior treatment psychological problems	0.393	0.000	0.195	0.000	0.257	0.035	0.128	0.030
No. people lived with[a]	−0.172	0.152	0.092	0.090	−0.015	0.898	0.058	0.690
Substance Dependence Index[a]	−0.204	0.040	0.107	0.060	−0.055	0.658	0.047	0.810
Substance Dependence Index[b]	−0.158	0.118	0.060	0.360	−0.051	0.687	0.043	0.760
Drug Crime Index, minus L3t	−0.334	0.001	0.134	0.000	−0.066	0.600	0.027	0.800
Living Risk Index	−0.364	0.000	0.156	0.000	−0.119	0.354	0.053	0.760
Vocational Risk Index	−0.002	0.982	0.153	0.000	0.085	0.493	0.081	0.480
Social Risk Index	−0.456	0.000	0.223	0.000	−0.134	0.313	0.103	0.280
Needle Frequency Index	−0.406	0.037	0.035	0.110	−0.618	0.069	0.024	0.320
Needle Problem Index	−0.067	0.549	0.009	0.780	−0.138	0.332	0.019	0.460
Sex Protection Ratio	0.038	0.703	0.038	0.820	−0.007	0.953	0.030	0.960

Table A.12—Continued

Variable	Unweighted				Weighted			
	Effect Size	P-value	KS Statistic	KS P-value	Effect Size	P-value	KS Statistic	KS P-value
Controlled Environment Index	−0.191	0.058	0.118	0.040	−0.066	0.579	0.060	0.660
General Satisfaction Index	0.257	0.015	0.141	0.000	0.063	0.618	0.076	0.590
Mental Health Treatment Index	−0.098	0.508	0.095	0.000	−0.501	0.211	0.083	0.150
Criminal Justice System Index	−0.628	0.000	0.331	0.000	−0.314	0.011	0.193	0.000
Training Problem Index	−0.239	0.016	0.130	0.020	−0.192	0.101	0.108	0.150
Substance Abuse Treatment Index	0.107	0.246	0.061	0.170	0.057	0.628	0.047	0.540
Substance Problem Index[a]	−0.195	0.052	0.159	0.000	−0.017	0.891	0.060	0.790
Substance Problem Index[b]	−0.092	0.358	0.053	0.620	0.045	0.708	0.057	0.770
Physical Health Treatment Index	0.083	0.478	0.123	0.010	0.153	0.132	0.122	0.060
Internal Mental Distress Index	−0.026	0.795	0.054	0.670	0.036	0.764	0.054	0.910
Environmental Risk Index	−0.332	0.002	0.169	0.000	−0.060	0.628	0.081	0.560
General Victimization Index	−0.300	0.003	0.160	0.010	−0.065	0.589	0.049	0.910
Personal Sources of Stress Index	0.025	0.801	0.039	0.680	0.090	0.438	0.051	0.740
Other Sources of Stress Index	0.085	0.390	0.064	0.250	0.108	0.362	0.075	0.360
Employment Problem Index	0.260	0.007	0.157	0.000	0.050	0.696	0.064	0.490
Employment Activity Index	0.395	0.000	0.204	0.000	0.145	0.238	0.093	0.350
Crime Violence Index	−0.594	0.000	0.258	0.000	−0.189	0.131	0.110	0.220
Illegal Activities Index	−0.181	0.067	0.107	0.090	−0.052	0.670	0.057	0.820
Substance Frequency Index	−0.495	0.000	0.192	0.000	−0.149	0.242	0.089	0.750
Current Withdrawal Index	−0.080	0.412	0.068	0.150	−0.056	0.632	0.058	0.450
Treatment Resistance Index	−0.364	0.000	0.147	0.000	−0.108	0.371	0.046	0.660
Treatment Motivation Index	−0.385	0.000	0.162	0.000	−0.137	0.252	0.074	0.350
Self-Efficacy Index	0.484	0.000	0.194	0.000	0.184	0.145	0.088	0.160
Problem Orientation Index	−0.043	0.666	0.038	0.450	0.043	0.722	0.037	0.620
Health Problem Index	0.582	0.000	0.345	0.000	0.247	0.034	0.149	0.020
Behavior Complexity Index	−0.173	0.088	0.119	0.050	−0.051	0.674	0.052	0.890
Emotional Problem Index	0.232	0.016	0.147	0.010	0.114	0.333	0.088	0.670
General Social Support Index	0.406	0.000	0.162	0.000	0.254	0.060	0.121	0.090
Training Activity Index	0.457	0.000	0.207	0.010	0.147	0.234	0.109	0.290
Recovery Environment Risk Index	−0.396	0.000	0.194	0.000	−0.158	0.212	0.099	0.370
Prior opiate use	−0.555	0.000	0.182	0.000	−0.242	0.059	0.080	0.120
Need for heroin treatment (self-reported)	NA	0.045	0.009	0.240	NA	0.144	0.009	0.150
Seizures/current withdrawal symptoms	−0.012	0.904	0.003	0.870	0.057	0.596	0.015	0.620

Table A.12—Continued

Variable	Unweighted				Weighted			
	Effect Size	P-value	KS Statistic	KS P-value	Effect Size	P-value	KS Statistic	KS P-value
Using daily	−0.151	0.118	0.070	0.110	−0.059	0.625	0.027	0.630
Using opioids[d]	−0.330	0.003	0.077	0.030	−0.087	0.482	0.020	0.420
Used in past two days	−0.404	0.000	0.126	0.000	−0.148	0.243	0.046	0.310
Substance use despite prior treatment	−0.590	0.000	0.146	0.000	−0.321	0.026	0.079	0.040
Acute health problems	0.631	0.000	0.308	0.000	0.301	0.015	0.147	0.000
High behavioral problems[a]	−0.315	0.003	0.115	0.000	−0.124	0.304	0.045	0.380
Days of victimization[c]	0.182	0.059	0.084	0.040	0.163	0.155	0.075	0.160
High victimization	−0.227	0.021	0.113	0.020	0.010	0.937	0.005	0.940
Current criminal justice involvement	−0.157	0.102	0.069	0.050	0.022	0.863	0.010	0.850
Total arrests[c]	−0.292	0.010	0.074	0.140	−0.100	0.464	0.047	0.510
Mental distress	0.103	0.290	0.050	0.290	0.015	0.904	0.007	0.890
High resistance	−0.580	0.000	0.108	0.000	−0.136	0.254	0.025	0.370
Low motivation	0.348	0.001	0.162	0.000	0.092	0.450	0.043	0.450
Low alc/drug use problem orientation	0.045	0.649	0.022	0.620	0.043	0.724	0.021	0.630
First high/intoxicated under age 15	−0.379	0.000	0.158	0.000	−0.244	0.033	0.102	0.050
Needle use[c]	−0.082	0.451	0.007	0.560	−0.154	0.299	0.013	0.510
In school	0.470	0.000	0.122	0.000	0.138	0.277	0.036	0.300
Employed	0.422	0.000	0.204	0.000	0.155	0.209	0.075	0.210
Homeless/runaway[a]	−0.213	0.043	0.058	0.060	−0.148	0.255	0.040	0.260
Family hist. of substance use	−0.151	0.118	0.070	0.080	−0.066	0.583	0.030	0.620
Weekly family problems[c]	0.249	0.010	0.121	0.000	0.195	0.100	0.095	0.060
Drunk/high most of day[d]	−0.614	0.000	0.243	0.000	−0.215	0.109	0.117	0.200
Tobacco Dependence Index[b,e]	0.094	0.345	0.074	0.380	0.054	0.672	0.065	0.740
Health Distress Index[a]	−0.036	0.716	0.040	0.630	−0.027	0.825	0.018	1.000
Homicidal-Suicidal Thought Index	0.201	0.034	0.085	0.010	0.160	0.155	0.067	0.200
Lifetime detox admissions	−0.533	0.028	0.033	0.070	−0.258	0.139	0.019	0.380
Attended AA or other self-help	−0.067	0.498	0.030	0.500	0.040	0.735	0.018	0.710
Last grade completed in school	0.385	0.000	0.175	0.000	0.131	0.299	0.052	0.710
Mention of alc as treatment need	0.099	0.302	0.036	0.200	0.154	0.165	0.056	0.170
Mention of marijuana as treatment need	−0.132	0.178	0.066	0.230	−0.196	0.101	0.098	0.120
Mention of cocaine as treatment need	−0.809	0.000	0.069	0.000	−0.275	0.099	0.023	0.140
Mention of opiates as treatment need	0.100	0.264	0.015	0.120	0.103	0.270	0.015	0.360
Mention of amph's as treatment need	−0.417	0.004	0.035	0.020	−0.153	0.231	0.013	0.350
Mention of other drugs as treatment need	0.159	0.081	0.039	0.010	0.111	0.314	0.027	0.250

Table A.12—Continued

Variable	Unweighted				Weighted			
	Effect Size	P-value	KS Statistic	KS P-value	Effect Size	P-value	KS Statistic	KS P-value
Controlled environment[c]	−0.174	0.087	0.134	0.010	−0.056	0.642	0.038	0.970
Currently in alc/drug treatment	−0.580	0.000	0.108	0.000	−0.286	0.063	0.053	0.060
Gender								
Male	−0.104	NA	0.045	0.190	−0.132	NA	0.057	0.220
Female	0.104	0.939	0.045	0.190	0.132	0.923	0.057	0.220
Race								
Am. Indian	−0.110	NA	0.009	0.410	−0.028	NA	0.002	0.700
Black	−0.111	NA	0.034	0.260	−0.205	NA	0.062	0.190
White	0.668	NA	0.269	0.000	0.326	1.000	0.131	0.020
Mexican	−0.826	0.996	0.120	0.000	−0.159	NA	0.023	0.310
Other race	−0.406	NA	0.105	0.010	−0.168	NA	0.044	0.180
Substance most likes								
Alcohol	0.115	NA	0.044	0.230	0.100	NA	0.038	0.420
Cannabis	0.124	NA	0.051	0.180	0.041	NA	0.017	0.700
Crack or cocaine	NA	NA	0.038	0.040	NA	NA	0.025	0.050
Opiates	0.002	NA	0.000	0.920	0.006	NA	0.001	0.680
Hallucinogens	−0.143	NA	0.021	0.210	−0.129	1.000	0.019	0.360
Amphetamines	−0.306	1.000	0.026	0.060	−0.025	NA	0.002	0.670
Other substance	NA	NA	0.009	0.250	NA	NA	0.010	0.100
Current living status								
House/apt	0.693	NA	0.141	0.000	0.323	NA	0.066	0.030
Friend/relative	−0.696	0.991	0.101	0.000	−0.435	0.997	0.064	0.020
Jail/correctional	−0.127	NA	0.019	0.260	0.041	NA	0.006	0.810
Other status	NA	NA	0.021	0.120	NA	NA	0.008	0.130

	N	Effective Sample Size	Average Effect Size	Max Effect Size	Average KS Statistic	Max KS Statistic	KS P-value
Unweighted	XXX[e]	XXX[e]	0.287	0.826	0.106	0.345	0.000
Weighted	XXX[e]	132.151	0.139	0.618	0.056	0.193	0.100

[a] Past year.

[b] Past month.

[c] Past 90 days.

[d] Weekly.

[e] Sample sizes censored in these tables to preserve program anonymity. For available sample sizes, see Table A.1.

Table A.13
Baseline Covariate Differences Between Program and Comparison Groups Before and After Weighting: Site J

Variable	Unweighted				Weighted			
	Effect Size	P-value	KS Statistic	KS P-value	Effect Size	P-value	KS Statistic	KS P-value
Age	−0.096	0.402	0.065	0.460	−0.073	0.619	0.051	0.750
Times received treatment for drug/alc	0.400	0.000	0.258	0.000	0.172	0.220	0.158	0.050
Prior treatment psychological problems	0.221	0.048	0.110	0.020	0.227	0.094	0.114	0.110
No. people lived with[a]	−0.295	0.021	0.134	0.040	−0.300	0.109	0.091	0.410
Substance Dependence Index[a]	0.746	0.000	0.309	0.000	0.347	0.015	0.165	0.010
Substance Dependence Index[b]	0.124	0.256	0.074	0.340	0.032	0.819	0.033	0.920
Drug Crime Index, minus L3t	0.184	0.093	0.115	0.050	0.183	0.146	0.121	0.120
Living Risk Index	0.119	0.274	0.077	0.350	−0.031	0.827	0.129	0.170
Vocational Risk Index	0.112	0.305	0.148	0.030	0.052	0.705	0.107	0.370
Social Risk Index	0.188	0.088	0.189	0.020	0.031	0.821	0.106	0.420
Needle Frequency Index	0.049	0.649	0.029	0.220	−0.035	0.791	0.019	0.810
Needle Problem Index	0.034	0.754	0.011	0.680	−0.157	0.336	0.036	0.220
Sex Protection Ratio	−0.133	0.225	0.083	0.320	−0.026	0.853	0.035	0.880
Controlled Environment Index	0.592	0.000	0.323	0.000	0.316	0.019	0.211	0.000
General Satisfaction Index	−0.356	0.001	0.195	0.000	−0.141	0.317	0.106	0.450
Mental Health Treatment Index	0.147	0.157	0.071	0.160	0.165	0.113	0.075	0.260
Criminal Justice System Index	1.128	0.000	0.388	0.000	0.156	0.254	0.068	0.300
Training Problem Index	0.256	0.026	0.121	0.050	0.078	0.611	0.077	0.640
Substance Abuse Treatment Index	0.317	0.003	0.294	0.000	0.210	0.075	0.197	0.010
Substance Problem Index[a]	0.754	0.000	0.281	0.000	0.322	0.028	0.144	0.060
Substance Problem Index[b]	0.094	0.393	0.079	0.390	0.022	0.871	0.054	0.900
Physical Health Treatment Index	−0.374	0.077	0.107	0.090	−0.219	0.276	0.112	0.110
Internal Mental Distress Index	0.371	0.001	0.227	0.000	0.140	0.308	0.132	0.330
Environmental Risk Index	0.199	0.071	0.123	0.090	0.029	0.833	0.042	1.000
General Victimization Index	0.539	0.000	0.292	0.000	0.261	0.068	0.160	0.060
Personal Sources of Stress Index	0.161	0.152	0.092	0.180	0.053	0.720	0.091	0.380
Other Sources of Stress Index	0.311	0.004	0.132	0.020	0.164	0.235	0.098	0.280
Employment Problem Index	−0.114	0.317	0.071	0.390	−0.028	0.847	0.068	0.420
Employment Activity Index	−0.257	0.023	0.139	0.040	−0.104	0.463	0.059	0.850
Crime Violence Index	0.116	0.285	0.086	0.410	0.048	0.713	0.060	0.920
Illegal Activities Index	−0.069	0.529	0.077	0.520	0.039	0.766	0.060	0.950
Substance Frequency Index	0.136	0.225	0.117	0.160	0.031	0.821	0.069	0.860

Table A.13—Continued

Variable	Unweighted				Weighted			
	Effect Size	P-value	KS Statistic	KS P-value	Effect Size	P-value	KS Statistic	KS P-value
Current Withdrawal Index	0.433	0.000	0.252	0.000	0.316	0.010	0.184	0.000
Treatment Resistance Index	0.328	0.003	0.133	0.040	0.141	0.298	0.086	0.460
Treatment Motivation Index	0.405	0.000	0.148	0.030	0.256	0.068	0.121	0.180
Self-Efficacy Index	−0.514	0.000	0.305	0.000	−0.177	0.211	0.118	0.150
Problem Orientation Index	0.179	0.105	0.088	0.090	0.071	0.605	0.038	0.820
Health Problem Index	−0.120	0.285	0.103	0.200	−0.105	0.489	0.045	1.000
Behavior Complexity Index	0.526	0.000	0.235	0.000	0.252	0.088	0.110	0.340
Emotional Problem Index	0.084	0.450	0.077	0.600	0.102	0.466	0.121	0.400
General Social Support Index	0.095	0.400	0.060	0.590	0.055	0.706	0.051	0.790
Training Activity Index	−0.198	0.072	0.134	0.080	−0.101	0.457	0.082	0.780
Recovery Environment Risk Index	0.536	0.000	0.271	0.000	0.222	0.095	0.105	0.580
Prior opiate use	0.617	0.000	0.308	0.000	0.517	0.000	0.259	0.000
Need for heroin treatment (self-reported)	NA	0.045	0.009	0.290	NA	0.139	0.018	0.210
Seizures/current withdrawal symptoms	0.347	0.001	0.138	0.000	0.262	0.031	0.104	0.030
Using daily	0.032	0.774	0.014	0.720	0.072	0.609	0.031	0.550
Using opioids[d]	0.269	0.012	0.109	0.000	0.179	0.154	0.072	0.130
Used in past two days	0.227	0.038	0.103	0.030	0.244	0.061	0.111	0.060
Substance use despite prior treatment	0.375	0.001	0.175	0.000	0.267	0.041	0.124	0.050
Acute health problems	−0.040	0.720	0.019	0.670	0.041	0.763	0.020	0.790
High behavioral problems[a]	0.455	0.000	0.226	0.000	0.195	0.155	0.096	0.180
Days of victimization[c]	0.210	0.056	0.099	0.030	0.123	0.352	0.058	0.340
High victimization	0.448	0.000	0.207	0.000	0.290	0.047	0.134	0.040
Current criminal justice involvement	0.861	0.000	0.190	0.000	0.186	0.182	0.041	0.220
Total arrests[c]	−0.038	0.724	0.055	0.390	−0.049	0.695	0.064	0.340
Mental distress	0.090	0.417	0.043	0.490	0.041	0.766	0.020	0.830
High resistance	0.290	0.007	0.119	0.000	0.132	0.326	0.054	0.370
Low motivation	−0.307	0.006	0.152	0.030	−0.259	0.062	0.129	0.100
Low alc/drug use problem orientation	−0.007	0.949	0.003	0.930	−0.015	0.915	0.007	0.940
First high/intoxicated under age 15	0.721	0.000	0.102	0.000	0.289	0.092	0.041	0.100
Needle use[c]	−0.026	0.818	0.003	0.840	−0.181	0.336	0.018	0.350
In school	−0.233	0.032	0.101	0.020	−0.166	0.221	0.072	0.200
Employed	−0.265	0.019	0.128	0.050	−0.115	0.415	0.056	0.320
Homeless/runaway[a]	0.324	0.003	0.138	0.000	0.137	0.314	0.058	0.230
Family hist. of substance use	0.443	0.000	0.151	0.000	0.209	0.164	0.071	0.190
Weekly family problems[c]	0.121	0.276	0.057	0.200	0.098	0.472	0.046	0.520
Drunk/high most of day[d]	0.234	0.034	0.167	0.000	0.118	0.375	0.082	0.720
Tobacco Dependence Index[b,e]	0.212	0.066	0.170	0.010	0.090	0.521	0.094	0.570

Table A.13—Continued

Variable	Unweighted				Weighted			
	Effect Size	P-value	KS Statistic	KS P-value	Effect Size	P-value	KS Statistic	KS P-value
Health Distress Index[a]	0.035	0.752	0.054	0.520	−0.008	0.953	0.033	0.950
Homicidal-Suicidal Thought Index	0.115	0.298	0.046	0.340	0.049	0.713	0.020	0.790
Lifetime detox admissions	0.045	0.744	0.040	0.040	−0.046	0.776	0.013	0.740
Attended AA or other self-help	0.508	0.000	0.254	0.000	0.222	0.113	0.111	0.110
Last grade completed in school	−0.168	0.138	0.080	0.340	0.046	0.738	0.063	0.670
Mention of alc as treatment need	−0.031	0.783	0.010	0.810	−0.097	0.526	0.032	0.520
Mention of marijuana as treatment need	−0.253	0.024	0.126	0.010	−0.274	0.049	0.137	0.060
Mention of cocaine as treatment need	0.104	0.341	0.028	0.230	0.063	0.616	0.017	0.700
Mention of opiates as treatment need	NA	0.014	0.013	0.160	NA	0.231	0.009	0.200
Mention of amph's as treatment need	0.404	0.000	0.146	0.000	0.268	0.037	0.097	0.020
Mention of other drugs as treatment need	0.034	0.761	0.007	0.760	−0.031	0.831	0.006	0.830
Controlled environment[c]	0.432	0.000	0.327	0.000	0.143	0.337	0.181	0.010
Currently in alc/drug treatment	0.568	0.000	0.269	0.000	0.310	0.025	0.147	0.010
Gender								
Male	−0.098	NA	0.042	0.340	−0.061	0.965	0.026	0.590
Female	0.098	0.943	0.042	0.340	0.061	NA	0.026	0.590
Race								
Am. Indian	0.164	NA	0.033	0.020	0.169	1.000	0.034	0.110
Black	−0.326	0.998	0.079	0.010	0.002	NA	0.000	1.000
White	−0.266	NA	0.133	0.020	−0.071	NA	0.035	0.650
Mexican	0.171	NA	0.063	0.070	−0.089	NA	0.033	0.580
Other race	0.268	NA	0.116	0.010	0.080	NA	0.034	0.500
Substance most likes								
Alcohol	−0.151	NA	0.046	0.170	−0.101	NA	0.031	0.480
Cannabis	−0.308	NA	0.149	0.000	−0.188	NA	0.091	0.170
Crack or cocaine	0.077	NA	0.015	0.520	−0.072	NA	0.014	0.600
Opiates	NA	NA	0.009	0.320	NA	NA	0.009	0.430
Hallucinogens	0.230	NA	0.067	0.000	0.152	NA	0.044	0.200
Amphetamines	0.381	1.000	0.130	0.000	0.301	1.000	0.102	0.000
Other substance	NA	NA	0.009	0.280	NA	NA	0.002	0.220
Current living status								
House/apt	−0.168	NA	0.068	0.080	−0.036	NA	0.015	0.820
Friend/relative	0.189	NA	0.068	0.040	0.128	NA	0.046	0.290
Jail/correctional	−0.304	0.996	0.031	0.100	−0.481	0.997	0.049	0.080
Other status	0.153	NA	0.030	0.030	0.086	NA	0.017	0.550

Table A.13—Continued

	N	Effective Sample Size	Average Effect Size	Max Effect Size	Average KS Statistic	Max KS Statistic	KS P-value
Unweighted	XXX[e]	XXX[e]	0.267	1.128	0.121	0.388	0.000
Weighted	XXX[e]	109.281	0.145	0.517	0.075	0.259	0.030

[a] Past year.

[b] Past month.

[c] Past 90 days.

[d] Weekly.

[e] Sample sizes censored in these tables to preserve program anonymity. For available sample sizes, see Table A.1.

Table A.14
Summary of Treatment Effects for All Facilities and All Outcomes

Facility	Recovery	Subst. Probs	Subst. Freq.	Illegal Acts	Emot. Probs	Days CE
Long Term Residential						
Site A	0.243	0.025	−0.008	0.244	0.692	−0.638
	(−0.133, 0.618)	(−0.458, 0.508)	(−0.513, 0.497)	(−0.292, 0.78)	(0.181, 1.202)	(−1.116, −0.16)
Site B	−0.019	0.082	0.113	−0.001	−0.005	−0.248
	(−0.26, 0.222)	(−0.248, 0.413)	(−0.194, 0.419)	(−0.288, 0.286)	(−0.261, 0.251)	(−0.52, 0.023)
Site C	−0.367	−6.714	−3.156	−0.571	−1.562	1.896
	(−0.818, 0.085)	(−9.817, −3.611)	(−4.576, −1.735)	(−1.893, 0.751)	(−2.351, −0.772)	(1.164, 2.628)
Short Term Residential						
Site D	0.245	−0.127	−0.286	0.166	0.176	−0.254
	(−0.078, 0.567)	(−0.506, 0.252)	(−0.649, 0.077)	(−0.196, 0.528)	(−0.172, 0.523)	(−0.595, 0.087)
Site E	−0.462	0.005	0.073	−0.015	−0.368	0.141
	(−0.865, −0.06)	(−0.301, 0.311)	(−0.243, 0.39)	(−0.324, 0.295)	(−0.607, −0.13)	(−0.139, 0.42)
Site F	−0.034	0.286	0.849	−0.802	0.158	−0.297
	(−0.948, 0.88)	(−0.73, 1.303)	(−0.322, 2.019)	(−1.743, 0.14)	(−0.864, 1.179)	(−1.435, 0.842)
Site G	0.176	0.096	0.092	0.122	0.29	−0.025
	(−0.114, 0.466)	(−0.168, 0.361)	(−0.194, 0.379)	(−0.175, 0.419)	(0.036, 0.544)	(−0.274, 0.224)
Outpatient						
Site H	−0.11	0.06	0.018	0.335	0.236	0.015
	(−0.351, 0.131)	(−0.192, 0.312)	(−0.245, 0.282)	(0.099, 0.571)	(0.022, 0.45)	(−0.205, 0.235)
Site I	0.212	0.003	−0.055	−0.088	0.222	0.06
	(−0.014, 0.439)	(−0.223, 0.228)	(−0.283, 0.173)	(−0.332, 0.156)	(−0.014, 0.458)	(−0.152, 0.273)
Site J	−0.048	−0.16	0.021	−0.213	−0.508	0.066
	(−0.348, 0.251)	(−0.464, 0.145)	(−0.34, 0.381)	(−0.571, 0.145)	(−0.897, −0.119)	(−0.263, 0.396)

Table A.15
Post-Hoc Power Calculations

Site	Power to Detect Small Effects[a]	Power to Detect Medium Effects[a]	Power to Detect Large Effects[a]
A	0.192	0.776	0.992
B	0.347	0.975	1.000
C	0.161	0.679	0.972
D	0.318	0.961	1.000
E	0.375	0.984	1.000
F	0.137	0.583	0.934
G	0.291	0.941	1.000
H	0.387	0.987	1.000
I	0.376	0.984	1.000
J	0.079	0.279	0.594
K	0.299	0.948	1.000

[a] Small effects are 0.20, medium effects are 0.50, and large effects are 0.80.

References

American Psychiatric Association. (1994). *Diagnostic and Statistical Manual of Mental Disorders* (4th ed.). Washington, D.C.: American Psychiatric Association.

Azrin, N. H., Donohue, B., Besalel, V. A., Kogan, E. S., and Acierno, R. (1994). Youth drug abuse treatment: A controlled outcome study. *Journal of Child and Adolescent Substance Abuse, 3*(3), 1–16.

Battjes, R. J., Sears, E. A., Katz, E. C., Kinlock, T. W., Gordon, M., and The Epoch Project Team. (2003). Evaluation of a group-based outpatient adolescent substance abuse treatment program. In S. J. Stevens and A. R. Morral (Eds.), *Adolescent Substance Abuse Treatment in the United States: Exemplary Models from a National Evaluation Study* (pp. 81–104). New York: Haworth Press.

Bluthenthal, R., Riehman, K. S., Jaycox, L. H., and Morral, A. R. (in press). Perspectives on therapeutic treatment from adolescent probationers. *Journal of Psychoactive Drugs.*

De Leon, G. (1999). Therapeutic communities. In P. J. Ott, R. E. Tarter, and R. T. Ammerman (Eds.), *Sourcebook on Substance Abuse: Etiology, Epidemiology, Assessment, and Treatment* (pp. 121–136). Needham Heights, Mass.: Allyn & Bacon.

Dennis, M. L. (1999). *Global Appraisal of Individual Needs (GAIN) Manual: Administration, Scoring and Interpretation.* Bloomington, Ill.: Lighthouse Publications. http://www.chestnut.org/li/gain.

Dennis, M. L., Dawud-Noursi, S., Muck, R. D., and McDermeit, M. (2003). The need for developing and evaluating adolescent treatment models. In S. J. Stevens and A. R. Morral (Eds.), *Adolescent Substance Abuse Treatment in the United States: Exemplary Models from a National Evaluation Study* (pp. 3–34). New York: Haworth Press.

Dennis, M., Godley, S. H., Diamond, G., Tims, F. M., Babor, T., Donaldson, J., Liddle, H., Titus, J. C., Kaminer, Y., Webb, C., Hamilton, N., and Funk, R. (2004). The Cannabis Youth Treatment (CYT) Study: Main findings from two randomized trials. *Journal of Substance Abuse Treatment, 27,* 197–213.

Dennis, M. L., McDermeit, M., and Funk, R. (June 23, 2002a). *Preliminary Data Tables and Charts For Cross-Site Analysis of the Adolescent Treatment Models Study (ATM/MASC).* Unpublished working document. Chestnut Health Systems.

Dennis M. L., Scott, C., Godley, M., and Funk, R. (1999). Comparisons of adolescents and adults by ASAM profile using GAIN data from the Drug Outcome Monitoring Study (DOMS): Preliminary data tables. Bloomington, Ill.: Chestnut Health Systems. http://www.chestnut.org/li/posters/asamprof.pdf (accessed June 10, 2003).

Dennis, M. L., Titus, J. C., Diamond, G., Donaldson, J., Godley, S. H., Tims, F. M., Webb, C., Kaminer, Y., Babor, T., Roebuck, M. C., Godley, M. D., Hamilton, N., Liddle, H., Scott, C. K., and CYT Steering Committee. (2002). The Cannabis Youth Treatment (CYT) xperiment: Rationale, study design, and analysis plans. *Addiction, 97,* Supl. 1, 84–97.

Efron, E., and Tibshirani, R. J. (1993). *An Introduction to the Bootstrap.* New York: Chapman & Hall.

Fishman, M., Clemmey, P., and Adger, H. (2003). Mountain Manor Treatment Center: Residential Adolescent Addictions Treatment Program. In S. J. Stevens and A. R. Morral (Eds.), *Adolescent Substance Abuse Treatment in the United States: Exemplary Models from a National Evaluation Study* (pp. 135–154). New York: Haworth Press.

Friedman, A. S. (1989). Family therapy vs. parent groups: Effects on adolescent drug abusers. *The American Journal of Family Therapy, 17*(4), 335–347.

Godley, M. D., Godley, S. H., Dennis, M. L., Funk, R., and Passetti, L. L. (2002). Preliminary outcomes from the assertive continuing care experiment for adolescents discharged from residential treatment. *Journal of Substance Abuse and Treatment, 23*(1), 21–32.

Godley, S. H., Risberg, R., Adams, L., and Sodetz, A. (2003). Chestnut Health Systems' Bloomington outpatient and intensive outpatient program for adolescent substance abusers. In S. J. Stevens and A. R. Morral (Eds.), *Adolescent Substance Abuse Treatment in the United States: Exemplary Models from a National Evaluation Study* (pp. 57–80). New York: Haworth Press.

Henggeler, S. W., Melton, G. B., and Smith, L. A. (1992). Family preservation using multisystemic therapy: An effective alternative to incarcerating serious juvenile offenders. *Journal of Consulting and Clinical Psychology, 60*(6), 953–961.

Hirano, K., Imbens, G., and Ridder, G. (2003). Efficient estimation of average treatment effects using the estimated propensity score. *Econometrica, 71,* 1161–1189.

Holland, P. W. (1986). Statistics and causal inference. *Journal of the American Statistical Association, 81,* 945–960.

Jainchill, N. (1997). Therapeutic communities for adolescents: The same and not the same. In G. De Leon (Ed.), *Community as Method: Therapeutic Communities for Special Populations and Special Settings* (pp. 161–178). Westport, Conn.: Praeger.

Jaycox, L. H., Morral, A. R., and Juvonen, J. (2003). Mental health and medical problems and service utilization among adolescent substance abusers. *Journal of the American Academy of Child and Adolescent Psychiatry, 42,* 311–318.

Liddle, H. A., Dakof, G. A., Parker, K., Diamond, G. S., Barrett, K., and Tejeda, M. (2001). Multidimensional family therapy for adolescent drug abuse: Results of a randomized clinical trial. *American Journal of Drug and Alcohol Abuse, 27,* 651–688.

Liddle, H. A., Rowe, C. L., Dakof, G. A., Ungaro, R. A., and Henderson, C. E. (2004). Early intervention for adolescent substance abuse: Pretreatment to posttreatment outcomes of a randomized clinical trial comparing multidimensional family therapy and peer group treatment. *Journal of Psychoactive Drugs, 36*(1), 49–63.

Little, R.J.A., and Rubin, D. B. (1987). *Statistical Analysis with Missing Data.* New York: Wiley.

McCaffrey, D. F., Ridgeway, G., and Morral, A. R. (2004). Propensity score estimation with boosted regression for evaluating causal effects in observational studies. *Psychological Methods, 9,* 403–425.

McGlynn, E. A., Asch, S. M., Adams, J., Keesey, J., Hicks, J., DeCristofaro, A., et al. (2003). The quality of health care delivered to adults in the United States. *New England Journal of Medicine, 348*(26), 2635–2645.

McLellan, A. T., McKay, J. R., Forman, R., Cacciola, J., and Kemp, J. (2005). Reconsidering the evaluation of addiction treatment: From retrospective follow-up to concurrent recovery monitoring. *Addiction, 100,* 447–458.

Mee-Lee, D., Shulman, G., Fishman, M., Gastfriend, D., and Griffith, J. (Eds.). (2001). *ASAM Patient Placement Criteria for the Treatment of Substance-Related Disorders (ASAM PPC-2R).* (2nd rev. ed.) Chevy Chase, Md.: American Society of Addiction Medicine, Inc.

Morral, A. R., Jaycox, L. H., Smith, W., Becker, K., and Ebener, P. (2003). An evaluation of substance abuse treatment services for juvenile probationers at Phoenix Academy of Lake View Terrace. In S. Stevens and A. R. Morral (Eds.), *Adolescent Substance Abuse Treatment in the United States: Exemplary Models from a National Evaluation Study* (pp. 213–234). New York: Haworth Press.

Morral, A. R., McCaffrey, D. F., and Chien, S. (2003). Measurement of adolescent drug use, *Journal of Psychoactive Drugs, 35,* 301–309.

Morral, A. R., McCaffrey, D. F., and Ridgeway, G. (2004). Effectiveness of community based treatment for substance abusing adolescents: 12-month outcomes from a case-control evaluation of a Phoenix academy. *Psychology of Addictive Behaviors, 18,* 257–268.

Orlando, M., Chan, K., and Morral, A. R. (2003). Retention of court-referred youths in residential treatment programs: Client characteristics and treatment process effects. *American Journal of Drug and Alcohol Abuse, 29,* 337–357.

Perry, P. D., Hedges, T. L., Douglas, C., Fusco, W., Carlini, K., Schneider, J., and Salerno, N. (2003). Dynamic Youth Community, Incorporated: A multiphase, step-down therapeutic community for adolescents and young adults. In S. J. Stevens and A. R. Morral (Eds.), *Adolescent Substance Abuse Treatment in the United States: Exemplary Models from a National Evaluation Study* (pp. 235–256). New York: Haworth Press.

Project Match Research Group. (1997). Matching alcoholism treatments to client heterogeneity: Project MATCH posttreatment drinking outcomes. *Journal of Studies on Alcohol, 58,* 7–29.

Ridgeway, G. (1999). The state of boosting. *Computing Science and Statistics, 31,* 172–181.

Ridgeway, G. (2004). GBM 1.1–2 package manual. http://cran.r-project.org/doc/packages/gbm.pdf (accessed April 28, 2004).

Riehman, K. S., Bluthenthal, R., Juvonen, J., and Morral, A. R. (2003). Exploring gender differences among adolescents in treatment: Findings from quantitative and qualitative analyses. *Journal of Drug Issues, Fall,* 865–896.

Rosenbaum, P. R., and Rubin, D. B. (1983). The central role of the propensity score in observational studies for causal effects. *Biometrika, 70,* 41–55.

Schell, T., Orlando, M., and Morral, A. R. (2005). Dynamic effects among patients' treatment needs, beliefs, and utilization: A prospective study of adolescents in drug treatment. *Health Services Research, 40,* 1128–1147.

Scott, C. K. (2004). A replicable model for achieving over 90% follow-up rates in longitudinal studies of substance abusers. *Drug and Alcohol Dependence, 74*(1), 21–36.

Shadish, W. R., Cook, T., and Campbell, D. (2002). *Experimental and Quasi-Experimental Designs for Generalized Causal Inference.* Boston: Houghton Mifflin Company.

Shane, P., Cherry, L., and Gerstel, T. (2003). Thunder Road Adolescent Substance Abuse Treatment Program. In S. J. Stevens and A. R. Morral (Eds.), *Adolescent Substance Abuse Treatment in the United States: Exemplary Models from a National Evaluation Study* (pp. 257–284). New York: Haworth Press.

Stevens, S. J., Estrada, B. D., Carter, T., Reinardy, L., Seitz, V., and Swartz, T. (2003). The Teen Substance Abuse Treatment Program: Program design, treatment issues, and client characteristics. In S. J. Stevens and A. R. Morral (Eds.), *Adolescent Substance Abuse Treatment in the United States: Exemplary Models from a National Evaluation Study* (pp. 37–56). New York: Haworth Press.

Stevens, S. J., Hasler, J., Murphy, B. S., Taylor, R., Senior, M., Barron, M., Garcia, P., and Powis, Z. (2003). La Cañada adolescent treatment program: Addressing issues of drug use, gender and trauma. In S. J. Stevens and A. R. Morral (Eds.), *Adolescent Substance Abuse Treatment in the United States: Exemplary Models from a National Evaluation Study* (pp. 183–212). New York: Haworth Press.

Stevens, S. J., and Morral, A. R. (Eds.). (2003). *Adolescent Substance Abuse Treatment in the United States: Exemplary Models from a National Evaluation Study.* New York: Haworth Press.

Stewart-Sabin, C., and Chaffin, M. (2003). Culturally competent substance abuse treatment for American Indian and Alaska Native youths. In S. J. Stevens and A. R. Morral (Eds.), *Adolescent Substance Abuse Treatment in the United States: Exemplary Models from a National Evaluation Study* (pp. 155–182). New York: Haworth Press.

Substance Abuse and Mental Health Services Administration (SAMHSA). (July, 2005). Measuring outcomes to improve services. *SAMHSA News, 4,* 3. http://alt.samhsa.gov/SAMHSA_News/VolumeXIII_4/article9.htm (accessed November 11, 2005).

Williams, R. J., Chang, S. Y., and Addiction Centre Research Group. (2000). A comprehensive and comparative review of adolescent substance abuse treatment outcome. *Clinical Psychology: Science and Practice, 7*(2), 138–166.

Winters, K. C. (1999). Treating adolescents with substance use disorders: An overview of practice issues and treatment outcomes. *Substance Abuse, 20*(4), 203–225.

Wooldridge, J. (2001). *Econometric Analysis of Cross Section and Panel Data.* Cambridge, Mass.: MIT Press.